Asthma in Practice

Fourth Edition

Mark Levy FRCGP and Sean Hilton MD FRCGP

Published by
The Royal College of General Practitioners
1999

Dedications

To my wife Celia
and parents Hymie and Rhoda Levy

and
To Nina, Adam and Thomas Hilton

© Royal College of General Practitioners

First edition 1987
Second edition 1992
Third edition 1993
Fourth edition 1999

Published by the Royal College of General Practitioners
14 Princes Gate
Hyde Park
London, SW7 1PU

Printed and bound by BSC Print Ltd, Wimbledon

ISBN 0 85084 243 3

CONTENTS

NOTE ABOUT THE AUTHORS

Mark Levy FRCGP graduated in Pretoria, South Africa in 1974 and emigrated to the United Kingdom in 1977. He has been a principal in general practice in Harrow since 1979, single-handed from 1986. Asthma is a particular interest of his; he has published papers on a variety of asthma management issues and has co-authored two books, one for people with asthma, *Asthma at Your Fingertips* and one for health professionals, *Shared Care in Asthma* and developed asthma himself in 1982. He was a trainer in general practice for 14 years and is currently active in the education of health professionals. A founder member of the General Practitioners in Asthma Group (GPIAG), Mark served as chairman from 1990 to 1993 and is currently the editor of the group's journal, *Asthma in General Practice*. He is a medical adviser to the Asthma Training Centre in Stratford-upon-Avon and a member of the Organisation of Care and the Therapy working groups of the UK Task Force on Asthma. He has been a member of both the National Asthma Campaign Education Committee and the working party that produced UK guidelines for the management of asthma in 1993 and 1997. Mark is also a reviewer for the Cochrane Airways Group.

Sean Hilton MD FRCGP DRCOG has been a principal in Kingston upon Thames since 1979, and is Dean of Undergraduate Medicine at St George's Hospital Medical School. His main clinical interest is in the management of asthma in primary care and he has published on management, audit and patient education in asthma. Sean was a general practitioner member of the British Thoracic Society/Royal College of Physicians working parties which produced guidelines for the management of asthma in 1990 and 1993. He is a Council member of the National Asthma Campaign and past Chairman of the National Asthma Campaign's Education Committee. He is also a Trustee of the National Asthma and Respiratory Training Centre in Warwick.

Balvinder Kaur MB BCh MRCP MFPHM is a lecturer in public health medicine at St George's Hospital Medical School and consultant in Public Health Medicine, West Midlands Regional Health Authority, Birmingham. Her main research interests are the epidemiology of asthma and other respiratory disorders.

Azeem Majeed MD MRCGP MFPHM is a medical epidemiologist at the Office for National Statistics and Senior Lecturer in the Department of General Practice at St George's Hospital Medical School. His main research interests are in prescribing in general practice and in health policy.

Ron Neville MD FRCGP DRCOG MBChB is a general practitioner in Dundee, Senior Lecturer in General Practice with the University of Dundee and Director of the GPIAG Research Unit. He has published on a number of subjects including: asthma and growth, asthma audit, computer assisted decision support and clinical outcomes.

Emma Sergeant RGN RSCN is Director of Communications at the National Asthma Respiratory Training Centre in Warwick. She is a qualified paediatric and adult nurse and has a NARTC Diploma in asthma care. She has contributed to NARTC publications, such as *Devices under Discussion* and *Ask the Experts* and various other medical press articles. She runs an asthma clinic with a register of 1,000 asthma patients.

PREFACE TO FOURTH EDITION

When chronic diseases occur they often impact severely on patients' lives. This should be of great concern to family doctors.

Asthma is a major chronic disease and its prevalence has increased markedly over recent decades. Despite this increase in prevalence death rates from asthma, which peaked in the 1960s and again in the late 1980s, have since fallen quite steadily and I venture to suggest that better management of asthma by primary care teams is a contributory factor.

In the early eighties underdiagnosis and management of asthma was a major problem and thanks to the pioneering work of such figures as Speight, Tudor Hart and Levy, this has now largely been reversed. National levels of diagnosis have now increased to 15% of children and about 7% of adults.

However, asthma continues to present formidable problems to practising clinicians. The early and correct identification of asthma is of extreme importance because of the vital therapeutic implications. Since the publication of the third edition of this book in 1993, knowledge of the epidemiology and pathogenesis of asthma has increased which, in turn, has led to improvement in the day-to-day management of patients.

The authors, Mark Levy and Sean Hilton, carried out major revision of their previous edition and incorporated all the relevant advances which are likely to improve both our understanding of the asthmatic process and the ways in which it can be managed effectively.

I am sure that this new edition will prove to be a valued resource for all clinicians caring for this important group of patients.

COLIN WAINE OBE FRCGP
Series Editor

1 Levy M (1986). Delay in diagnosing asthma – is the nature of general practice to blame? *Journal of the Royal College of General Practitioners* **36**: 52-53

2 Speight ANP (1978). Is childhood asthma being under diagnosed and under treated? *BMJ* **2**: 331-332

3 Tudor Hart J (1986). Wheezing in young children: problems of measurement and management. *Journal of the Royal College of General Practitioners* **36**(288): 78-8

· 1 ·

INTRODUCTION

Asthma is one of the commonest and most important conditions encountered in general practice in the United Kingdom. It is the commonest chronic condition of children and it makes a major impact on medical, domestic, school and industrial life. There are over three million people suffering from asthma symptoms during the course of any one year in the UK – more than one million of them children – and the majority of these will consult their general practitioner because of these symptoms at least once during that year. There is a wide spectrum of severity and much evidence to show that consulting behaviour is not necessarily related to that severity. Despite improvements in care in recent years, there currently are approaching 100,000 hospital admissions each year for acute asthma, and nearly 2,000 deaths recorded as due to asthma each year in the UK. These numbers are considerably greater than in the 1950s, when the first of the modern therapies - which are so highly effective - became available. Paradoxically, asthma has become more prevalent and more problematic as our understanding of the disease and its treatments has improved.

Asthma gives rise to enormous financial costs: costs not only to the National Health Service and the Department of Social Security but also to the nation as a whole in terms of lost productivity. These costs were estimated as approaching £1 billion in 1990, and probably now exceed that figure.

National surveys of asthmatics have drawn responses from over 50,000 people from all regions in the UK (Action Asthma 1991, Impact of asthma survey 1996, National Asthma Campaign and Allen & Hanburys). While only 6% of the sample felt that their asthma was severe, a much higher proportion reported symptomatology of a severe nature. More than half reported having symptoms every day, 70% had symptoms weekly or more often and 19% were waking every night. Two thirds reported that asthma was exerting either moderate or major effects on their qual-

ity of life, and 1 in 25 felt that asthma had total control over their life. Only 3% of the total were solely under hospital care, with the vast majority receiving community care, either from the general practitioner alone (65% of cases) or as shared care between the general practitioner and the hospital (23%). Of perhaps greater significance was the finding that 9% had received no medical care at all in the preceding year and yet their symptoms were not significantly milder than those receiving care.

The most important point to be underlined by the findings of these large surveys is the apparent mismatch between patients' and professionals' expectations of treatment. One third of those patients woken three or more times a week by symptoms viewed their asthma as 'not very' or 'not at all' severe, and almost half of those waking once or twice a week felt the same. It is unlikely that those treating the asthma would have taken the same view, yet patients seemed to exhibit a surprisingly uncomplaining attitude towards quite severe levels of symptoms. Other surveys have also highlighted a reluctance amongst quite severely affected patients to 'trouble' their doctors.

HISTORY OF ASTHMA

Asthma has been described, though not explicitly, in medical writings since the ancient civilisations of Egypt and China, as far back as the third millennium. In a famous sixteenth century case history, the Paduan physician Cardan travelled from Italy to treat the asthma of Hamilton, Archbishop of St Andrew's, Scotland. One feature of the treatment he recommended was the avoidance of influences now familiar to us as trigger factors: cold air, emotional stress and feather pillows. In 1698 Floyer, himself an asthmatic, published *A Treatise of the Asthma* in which he differentiated the 'continued' variety of dyspnoea from the 'periodic'.

Although there have been detailed and elegant descriptions of the clinical features of asthma for centuries, there seems to have been some sort of transformation in its natural history within the past one hundred years. As recently as 1897, in his textbook *The Principles and Practice of Medicine*, the great physician Osler made the following statement:

"We have no knowledge of the morbid anatomy of true asthma. Death during the acute attack is unknown. In long standing cases the lesions are those of chronic bronchitis and emphysema."

Has the nature of asthma changed?

From a condition described by Osler as a 'neurotic affliction', asthma has become a major cause of early and preventable death; a killer of more than 2,000 people each year in the United Kingdom. How has this occurred?

There must be many factors involved – if these could be identified and pulled together, it would surely go a long way towards reversing the toll exacted by asthma. Of course, there has been a great increase in life expectancy throughout the twentieth century, as a result of improvements in socioeconomic conditions and the eclipse of former major killers such as tuberculosis and other infectious diseases. Under these circumstances other causes of death inevitably become more prominent. There has also been enormous environmental change, particularly in the industrial centres of the country. The Clean Air Act of the 1950s led to great reductions in deaths from chronic obstructive bronchitis, but more recent environmental perils seem to threaten worsening conditions for those with asthma. The sad sight of the athlete Steve Ovett succumbing to acute asthma in the ozone filled smog of the Los Angeles Olympics of 1988 was perhaps the most striking example of the potential for more modern atmospheric pollution to give rise to respiratory problems. Intensive research since that time seems to have ruled out modern urban pollution as the *cause* of changes in the prevalence or natural history of asthma, but it does play a role in exacerbating pre-existing asthma.

For the first time in thousands of years a wide range of effective treatments for asthma has become available - at a time when the condition has exerted its greatest effects on mortality and mor-

---

Possible explanations for an increase in the severity of asthma include:

- an increase in the prevalence of asthma itself

- an increase in the severity of asthma amongst those suffering from it

- (most worryingly) long-term harmful effects of treatments which confer short-term benefits

---

bidity. This is a rich irony which provides a great challenge to all those involved in its management.

It seems likely from a number of international studies that the first explanation is at least partly responsible. Among the hypotheses put forward to explain an increasing prevalence, the most plausible is the suggestion that people are becoming more easily sensitised to allergens in the home and wider environment, and to other factors which have increased in prevalence, most notably pollutants of all sorts (see Chapter 3). Many experienced clinicians feel that the severity of asthma has worsened in recent years amongst those admitted to hospital. Once more, changing environmental factors could reasonably account for this.

Of much greater concern must be the suggestion that certain of the accepted medical treatments may actually have an insidious adverse effect on asthma. Some studies, notably those looking at the effects of beta agonist drugs on metabolism and bronchial reactivity, raised this spectre in a most unsettling way (*Lancet*, 1990); and the safety of beta agonists has been the focus of much research in recent years. There now seems to be little doubt that the epidemic of asthma deaths which occurred in New Zealand during the 1980s was directly related to the availability and use of a particular beta agonist, fenoterol.

ASTHMA CARE IN GENERAL PRACTICE

Successful asthma care requires a high index of suspicion for diagnosis, followed by carefully planned management, with a continuing and co-operative relationship between practice team and patient (and/or parents). A number of features make asthma pre-eminently suitable for care in general practice:

- its chronicity, which makes continuity of care desirable

- the fact that it affects all age groups

- the importance of family histories in diagnosis and management

- the importance of the environment in which the patient lives and works

- the fact that it is common: most studies suggest prevalence figures of around 5% (and rising) of the population overall

- it lends itself to all facets of primary care: prevention; diagnosis; acute and continuing care; and teamwork

- it can be managed effectively without complicated technology or specialist skills

However, although asthma is a condition ideally suited to management in general practice, much published research in the past had shown it to be underdiagnosed and undertreated in this setting (Anderson et al., 1981; Speight et al., 1983; Levy and Bell, 1984).

In 1981, an unsigned editorial in the *Journal of the Royal College of General Practitioners* (RCGP, 1981) called for a revolution in the GP management of asthma. The article encouraged a more pro-active approach to diagnosis and regular supervision of care with preventive therapy, allied to better monitoring of respiratory function. Over the past 10 to 15 years it is probably fair to say that the changes in asthma care have been close to revolutionary. The box below shows some of the major developments since the mid 1980s.

These contractual and service changes, allied with multiple educational initiatives for general practitioners, and major training programmes for practice nurses (the latter spearheaded by the extraordinary success of the National Asthma and Respiratory Training Centre NARTC), have led to the revolution. There is accumulating evidence that improvements in the process of general practice asthma care are having a beneficial effect on asthma mortality and morbidity. However, much remains to be achieved.

In this latest edition of *Asthma in Practice*, the influence of these changes on organisation of asthma care will be discussed. The book contains a number of major revisions, reflecting advances in our understanding of asthma, in addition to the greatly changed primary care environment in which general practice teams deliver care.

Influences on asthma care in general practice since 1980s:

GP contract including payment for health promotion clinics (1990)

Chronic Disease Management Programme for asthma and diabetes (1993)

Major involvement of practice nurses in organised asthma care (1987 onwards)

Publication of national and local guidelines for asthma management (from 1987)

NHS reforms, including GP fundholding, commissioning and most recently primary care groups (during 1990s)

Peak flow meters available on prescription (December 1990)

A Chronic
Inflammatory Condition

Introduction

Traditionally asthma was regarded as a disease process involving episodic bronchoconstriction, and treated as if it were a series of discrete, acute illnesses. The literature suggests that doctors were resistant to accepting that asthmatic patients were actually suffering from a chronic inflammatory process requiring long-term management.

This chapter summarises current thoughts on the underlying pathology of asthma, and the inflammatory process and its likely relationship to bronchial hyper-reactivity (BHR). The clinical implications of these processes and the conclusion reached is that asthma should be approached as a chronic condition.

It is hoped that this chapter will stimulate members of primary care teams to re-examine their approach to the management of patients with asthma and institute changes where appropriate.

Structure and function

Distal to the main bronchi, the protective arrangement of cartilage and smooth muscle on airway patency (whereby the smooth muscle is attached only between the posterior tips of an anterior cartilage 'crescent'), is lost. Cartilage disappears completely from the airway wall by the sixth or seventh generation of branches.

The airways' lining is a pseudo-stratified ciliated columnar epithelium. There are many submucosal glands, more abundant in the larger bronchi, and they contribute to the normal airway secretions along with tissue fluid and epithelial exudates.

Innervation of the airways is by the autonomic system: both sympathetic, with alpha and beta adrenergic receptors, and parasympathetic, with vagal and cholinergic receptors. Stimulation of sympathetic receptors leads to bronchodilatation by relaxation of the musculature, whereas parasympathetic stimulation leads to bronchoconstriction. These properties are important in drug treatment.

An unidentified number of chemical mediators, including leucotrienes and vasoactive intestinal peptide (VIP), are also involved in the control of airway function.

Pathogenesis

The clinical features of asthma result from pathological changes in the state of the intra-pulmonary airways as a result of abnormal sensitivity, usually termed bronchial hyper-reactivity. The muscle of the bronchial walls becomes hypertrophied. Distal to the major bronchi, as the cartilage in the walls disappears completely; the airway becomes susceptible to occlusion by contraction of this muscle. This component of airways narrowing may accurately be described as 'bronchospasm', but is not the only, nor necessarily the most important component.

There is also a characteristic inflammatory cell infiltrate in the mucosal, submucosal and smooth muscle layers. The most numerous of these cells is the eosinophil, but also found in varying numbers are neutrophils, macrophages, mast cells and plasma cells. All contain a number of putative chemical mediators of the 'asthmatic response'. There is an increase in luminal secretions, containing mucus, eosinophils, desquamated epithelial cells and other proteins and tissue exudates, all of which plug smaller airways. The pathological effects of asthma on small airways make take appreciably longer to resolve than those involving larger airways.

It is vital, therefore, not to consider asthma as a condition merely caused by 'bronchospasm', but to take account of the three main components of airway narrowing: muscle constriction, mucosal swelling due to oedema and infiltration, and increased intraluminal secretions.

NATURE OF THE ASTHMATIC RESPONSE

The sequence of events which follows the exposure of asthmatics to allergens have been studied both *in vitro* and *in vivo*. This has been clearly summarised by Djukanovic and colleagues (1989). There is a two-stage process in the airways following exposure to an allergen: an immediate and a late asthmatic response (see Figure 2.1). The immediate response results in intense bronchoconstriction within 30 minutes of exposure, presumably as a result of the release by inflammatory cells (eg mast cells and macrophages) of preformed mediators such as histamine, chemotactic factors, and newly formed mediators such as prostaglandins, leukotrienes and platelet-activating factor (PAF). A comprehensive report of expert opinions on inflammatory processes in asthma, suggests that the evidence for involvement of inflammatory cells (many of which produce mediators) in the pathogenesis of asthma is circumstantial (Holgate, 1989). Although cells like eosinophil and neutrophil leucocytes, mast cells, macrophages and epithelial cells are found in bronchioalveolar lavage specimens, their function could possibly be to repair the inflammation.

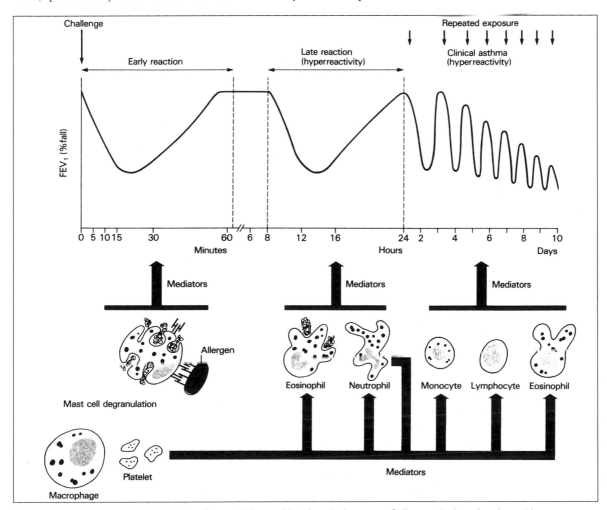

Figure 2.1 Schematic representation of the cellular and biochemical events of allergen-induced early and late asthmatic reactions and clinical asthma

Source: First published in Holgate ST (1986) and Cochrane GM (1987). Reproduced with permission of the author and publisher, Sutton, Reed Healthcare Communications.

The last ten years has seen a massive increase in research into the basic mechanisms underlying the disease process. A wide range of chemicals and mediators is involved in the process. In a review of the cellular and mediator basis of asthma Holgate concluded that the *"variable and complex clinical presentations of asthma are the consequences of an interplay between T-lymphocyte mediated inflammation, tissue destruction and remodelling"* (Holgate, 1997). No longer are one or two key cells or humoral agents such as mast cells and histamine viewed as central to the asthma disease mechanism, but a wide range of substances involved in complex interrelationships. These include:

- adenosine
- chemotactic factors
- cytokines
- endothelin
- eosinophil granule proteins
- lipid derived chemicals, including important mediators, such as:
  1. cyclo-oxygenase products (eg prostaglandins)
  2. lipoxygenase products (eg leucotrienes)
  3. platelet activating factor
- neuropeptides
- nitric oxide

See Chapter 5 for an understanding of the mechanisms which lead the way towards newer and better therapeutic options for the management of asthma.

Bronchial hyper-reactivity

The term bronchial hyper-reactivity refers to the abnormal sensitivity of the airways to nonspecific bronchoconstrictor agents (Scadding, 1983). Bronchial hyper-reactivity has long been accepted as a cardinal feature of asthma and because of its nonspecific nature, attacks may be caused by many factors known to be triggers of asthma. Bronchial hyper-reactivity is common to skin test positive (atopic) and skin test negative (non-atopic) asthmatics, and therefore it cannot be used to differentiate between them. Moreover, it is also found in a number of other respiratory conditions: chronic bronchitis, cystic fibrosis, following croup in children and viral infections in normal subjects, in extrinsic allergic alveolitis, and in patients with occupational-induced asthma (Melillo et al., 1986). Regular smokers have a high prevalence of bronchial hyper-reactivity. Other conditions associated with bronchial hyper-reactivity in children include bronchiectasis, chronic simple cough, infantile bronchiolitis, and even near drowning in early childhood (Silverman, 1985).

Thus, it can be seen that bronchial hyper-reactivity is not a specific marker for asthma. Overall, however, its prevalence is higher in asthmatics than in any other group (Melillo et al. 1986).

Confirmation of the presence of bronchial hyper-reactivity is made by testing the individual patient's response to an inhaled agent, usually from a nebuliser. Conventionally, this is quantified by the dose required to reduce the FEV_1 by 20%. Two methods have been in common use since the late 1970s. One involves a timed administration of an agent (Cockcroft et al., 1977) and the other a counted number of doses of an agent (Yen et al., 1983). The two agents most commonly used to study bronchial hyper-reactivity are methacholine and histamine, but cold air and exercise are other examples. When estimating prevalence, care needs to be taken to exclude those people with temporary changes in reactivity, such as those caused by acute viral infections.

The mechanisms responsible for inducing bronchial hyper-reactivity have been the subject of debate for the past 20 years. Smoking appears to induce persistent bronchial hyper-reactivity and the extent to which this develops is often related to the duration of smoking. Prospective studies of people who have given up smoking have shown a halt in the otherwise progressive increase in bronchial hyper-reactivity. It has been suggested that in view of the high occurrence of bronchial hyper-reactivity in patients with genetic disorders such as cystic fibrosis and Kartagener's syndrome, there may be an inherited component. Some studies suggest a higher prevalence of bronchial hyper-reactivity in people living in rural compared with urban areas (Woolcock et al., 1987; Iverson et al., 1989). Theoretically there are many complex factors which may contribute to increased hyper-responsiveness including the calibre of the airways, airways smooth muscle autonomic stimuli and non-adrenergic non-cholinergic stimulation (Raffery and Holgate, 1987).

Inflammation

The role of inflammation in the development and maintenance of bronchial hyper-reactivity has not been fully explained, but it is likely to be very significant. It has been suggested that once initiated, the inflammation persists and as a result acts as a stimulus to bronchial hyper-reactivity (Chung, 1986; Hargreave, 1988). It is worth noting that the inflammation of asthma has even been found in the airways of asymptomatic asthma patients between attacks (Chung, 1986).

Clinical relevance

The clinical manifestation of bronchial hyper-reactivity is likely to be cough, wheeze and chest tightness or difficulty in breathing. Patients with no increase in bronchial hyper-reactivity seldom have symptoms of asthma, and the degree of hyper-reactivity has been shown to correlate closely with both clinical severity and the need for rescue drug usage in acute asthma (Makino, 1966; Cockcroft et al., 1977; Juniper et al., 1981; Holgate, 1989).

Asthmatic patients who are asymptomatic on treatment, or are in remission, need to know that many factors can trigger underlying bronchial hyper-reactivity (twitchy airways) with consequent return of asthma symptoms. Very often these first 'breakthrough' symptoms will occur at night; sometimes they will come on gradually and often they are atypical (that is, wheeze may

not be present, see Chapter 4). Many patients become used to these continuing symptoms of asthma, and accept them as part of 'normal' life. Often, with identification and appropriate treatment they can be abolished.

All asthma experts now agree that therapy should be directed much more towards the underlying inflammation that represents the fundamental pathological process of asthma.

A BALANCED APPROACH

In view of the inflammatory nature of asthma general practitioners should reconsider their approach to the management of asthmatic patients. While remaining alert to asthmatics as yet undiagnosed in the practice, they also need to reappraise their method of following up and reassessing those already diagnosed. Perhaps some lessons can be taken from the more methodical approach to 'acknowledged' chronic diseases such as diabetes and hypertension. The success of nurse-run asthma clinics and the introduction of the Chronic Disease Management Programme have helped to put asthma high on the practice agenda for action, thereby ensuring regular follow-up and proper surveillance (see Chapter 9). Each patient needs to be monitored frequently, by self-assessment and attendance at the practice or outpatients.

Much has been written about undertreatment and underdiagnosis of asthma, but we feel that patients also tend to be under-assessed. This under-assessment applies to all patients with previously diagnosed asthma, wherever they receive their care, and occurs as a result of failure to appreciate the chronicity of asthma. The implications of this approach to asthma are dealt with in Chapters 5 and 6.

· 3 ·

HAS ASTHMA CHANGED?

INTRODUCTION

The prevalence and severity of asthma are thought to have increased substantially in recent decades. Major changes in the patterns of management of asthma have included greater use of prophylactic medication and an increase in hospital admission rates. In this chapter, some of these changes are examined in more detail. The objective is to give members of the primary care team sufficient background information against which they can compare their own practice.

DISEASE DEFINITION

One problem with epidemiological surveys of the incidence and prevalence of asthma is the absence of an agreed case definition; this leads to problems comparing the results of different studies (Strachan DP, 1995a). In previous epidemiological studies, three different methods have generally been used to diagnose asthma (see Table 3.1).

Some studies have used a 'diagnosis' of asthma by a doctor. In studies of health care utilisation rates, such as trends in hospital admission rates or general practice consultation rates, this will be the only method of diagnosis available. The main problem with this is that there is great variation between doctors in their propensity to diagnose asthma. For this reason, most epidemiological studies have used 'symptoms' to diagnose

asthma. The advantages of using symptoms, such as the presence of wheeze to label children as asthmatics, in epidemiological studies are:

- this method is independent of variations in doctors' preferences to diagnose asthma
- the full range of asthma symptoms can be investigated

Using symptoms of wheezing to diagnose children as having asthma does make the assumption that all wheezing is due to asthma, which is not always the case. Finally, some studies have used 'bronchial hyper-reactivity' (see Chapter 2) to define asthma. However, this technique is too invasive and labour-intensive for routine use in epidemiological studies.

INCIDENCE

Incidence is defined as the number of new events or cases of a disease that develop in a population during a specified period of time. It gives an estimate of the probability or risk that an individual will develop a disease during a specified period of time. As discussed above, to some extent the incidence of asthma depends on how asthma is defined and measured. In the National Child Development Study, a cohort of 16,883 children born in March 1958 were followed up at 7, 11, 16 and 23 years (Anderson HR et al., 1992).

Case definition	Advantages	Disadvantages
Diagnosis of asthma by a doctor	High specificity (few false positives)	Low sensitivity (many false negatives)
Symptom-based (eg presence of wheeze)	Simple and independent of diagnostic fashion	May not be specific for asthma (eg some false positives due to bronchitis). Some cases of asthma may present with a chronic cough
Airway reactivity (eg to test challenges)	An objective measurement	Not specific for asthma. Sensitivity, specificity and repeatability of tests vary

Table 3.1 Definitions of cases of asthma used in epidemiological surveys

Age group (years)	0-7	8-11	12-16	17-23
Number of new cases	1311	261	201	291
Number of children in study	7225	5914	5653	5452
Cumulative incidence (number of new cases by final year of age group per 100 children)	18.2	21.8	24.5	28.6
Average annual incidence (number of new cases per 100 children per year)	2.6	1.1	0.7	0.8

Table 3.2 Incidence of 'attacks of asthma or wheezy bronchitis' in Britain: The 1958 National Child Development Study

Source: Based on information found in the following article: Anderson et al., 1992.

Table 3.2 reveals that the incidence of asthma (defined as asthma attacks or wheezy bronchitis) was highest in children aged 0 to 7 years. By the age of 23 years, over one quarter of the children in the study had suffered at least one attack of asthma or 'wheezy bronchitis'.

PREVALENCE

Prevalence is defined as the number of cases of a disease in a population at any one time and is expressed as a rate, usually per 1,000 people, or as a percentage. As with incidence, the prevalence of asthma can be influenced by the case definition and the method of data collection. Hence, care needs to be taken when comparing the results of different surveys. National estimates for the prevalence of asthma and wheeze are shown in Table 3.3.

Criterion for defining asthma	Percentage of children
Wheeze within the last 12 months	12-15
Diagnosis of asthma	8-10
Requiring regular treatment	4-6
Persistent wheeze	4
Severe acute attacks of asthma	1
Disabling disease	1-2

Table 3.3 Prevalence of wheeze and asthma in Britain

Source: Based on information found in the following article: Anderson et al., 1994a.

Between 8 and 10% of children have a current diagnosis of asthma, of which about half require regular treatment. Around one percent of children suffer from severe attacks of asthma or from disabling disease.

GEOGRAPHICAL VARIATIONS

A study published in 1998 (ISAAC UK) measured the prevalence of asthma symptoms in 27,500 12 to 14 year old children, in 93 schools across Britain (Kaur et al., 1998). They found that about one third of 12 to 14 year olds had suffered from wheezing in the previous 12 months. There was little geographical variation in prevalence. Symptoms of asthma seemed equally common in urban and rural areas, and in the different NHS regions of England. There were also only small differences between England, Scotland and Wales. For most symptoms of asthma, there was less than a 1.3 fold variation between areas with the highest and lowest prevalence. Previous national studies also found little variation in the prevalence of asthma in 11 year olds and 5 to 17 year olds in Britain (Strachan DP et al., 1990; Strachan DP et al., 1994). The variation between different areas of Britain is substantially lower than the 20-fold global variation in the prevalence of asthma symptoms found in the ISAAC study. In this study, the prevalence of asthma and other atopic disorders was found to be much higher in Britain than in the majority of the 56 countries in the ISAAC study (ISAAC Steering Committee, 1998).

TIME TRENDS

Four city-based and two national studies of time trends in the prevalence of asthma all show an increase in prevalence (Whincup PH et al., 1993; Anderson HR et al., 1994b; Omran M et al., 1996; Burr et al., 1989; Strachan DP et al., 1990; Rona et al., 1995). The studies differ in the age groups they covered, the time period of the study, and the definitions of asthma used. Although these problems make it difficult to compare the results of the studies, the findings (see Tables 3.4 and 3.5) are consistent with a 20-30% relative increase in the prevalence of wheezing over the last 25 years and a two-fold increase in the prevalence of diagnosed asthma.

	10 towns	Croydon	Aberdeen	Cardiff
Age group (years)	6-7	7-8	8-11	1?
Time periods	1966-1970	1978–1991	1964–1994	1973–1988
Definition of asthma	Wheeze ever	Wheeze in last 12 months	Wheeze in last 3 years	Wheeze in last 12 months
Prevalence				
at start (%)	17.8	11.1	10.4	9.8
at end (%)	23.1	12.8	25.4	15.2
Definition of asthma	Persistent wheeze	Wheeze in past month	Diagnosed asthma	Asthma ever
Prevalence				
at start (%)	3.9	3.5	4.1	5.5
at end (%)	6.1	7.8	19.6	12.0

Table 3.4 City-based surveys of trends in the prevalence of childhood asthma and wheeze in Britain

Source: Based on information found in the following articles - Anderson et al., 1994a; Burr et al., 1989; Omran and Russell, 1996; Whincup et al., 1993.

	1958 & 1970 NCDS	National Study of Health & Growth	National Study of Health & Growth
Area	**Britain**	**England**	**Scotland**
Time period	1958 and 1970	1982 and 1992	1982 and 1992
Age group (years)	1958 - 7 and 16 1970 - 5 and 16	5-11	5-11
Asthma definition	1958 - Asthma or wheezy bronchitis 1970 - Wheezing in the last year	Asthma attacks	Asthma attacks
Prevalence at start (%)	9.0 (age 7) 3.8 (age 16)	4.2 (boys) 2.7 (girls)	3.9 (boys) 2.1 (girls)
Prevalence at end (%)	9.9 (age 5) 6.5 (age 16)	11.8 (boys) 7.0 (girls)	10.3 (boys) 5.9 (girls)

Table 3.5 National surveys of trends in the prevalence of childhood asthma and wheeze in Britain

Source: Based on information found in the following articles: Strachan et al., 1990; Rona et al., 1995.

RISK FACTORS AND AETIOLOGY

The identification of possible risk factors is the first key step in determining the aetiology of a disease. A risk factor is a characteristic that is present more commonly among persons who have (or later develop) a disease than those who do not.

The best available evidence about the aetiology of asthma comes from cohort and prevalence studies. The strongest risk factors appear to be genetic (see Table 3.6).

Moderate (relative risk greater than 2)	Comment
1. Genetic	Family history of asthma or atopy
2. Atopy	Hay fever, eczema, positive skin prick tests
3. Chest infections	Respiratory syncytial virus, pneumonia or whooping cough in childhood
4. Smoking (adults)	

Weak (relative risk between 1 and 2)	
1. Male sex	
2. Passive smoking	Exposure in early childhood years
3. Mother under 20 years of age	

Inconclusive	
1. Exposure to allergens	Domestic pets
2. Chemical exposure	Occupational
3. Air pollution	Small effect only from rises in pollutants
4. Socioeconomic factors	Little impact on prevalence after 5 years of age
5. Month of birth	Via early infections
6. Intra-uterine factors	Maternal smoking, exposure to allergens

Table 3.6 Risk factors for asthma

There is also compelling evidence that environmental factors have been influential in the recent increase in the prevalence of childhood asthma:

- the time over which the increase has occurred is too short for a genetic shift in populations
- migrants appear to acquire the prevalence level of their host area
- the concordance for asthma in monozygotic twins is only about 30%
- in asthmatic patients, many of the factors provoking an asthma attack are clearly environmental

In children, upper respiratory tract infections are the commonest factors triggering an acute attack of asthma (see Table 3.7). Other risk factors currently being examined include: dietary; infection and hygiene; foetal and early childhood; and the indoor environment.

Trigger factor	Percentage of children with wheeze who experienced episodes provoked by factor
Colds	95
Season	65
Weather	56
Exercise	53
Tobacco smoke	38
Excitement or emotional upset	35
Animals	32
Plants, grass	31
House dust	19
Foods	6

Table 3.7 Factors provoking wheezing episodes in children

Source: Based on information found in the following article: Anderson et al., 1994a.

Influence on Family Structure

There appears to be a negative association between family size and the prevalence of atopic disorders such as hay fever and asthma (Strachan DP, 1995b). The prevalence of atopic disorders is highest in firstborn children and lowest in children with several older siblings. Hence, the position of a child in the household appears to influence the risk of developing atopy. The apparent protective effect of older siblings may be seen as an example of biological 'programming'. The precise nature of this programming remains uncertain, but one hypothesis is that allergic sensitisation can be prevented by infections acquired during early childhood. Other people living in the household often transmit infections to young children, particularly older siblings attending schools or playgroups. This hypothesis is supported by the low prevalence of hay fever among children from poorer families living in rented accommodation or sharing household amenities with other families. Such living conditions may expose children to unhygienic lifestyles or household conditions that promote the spread of infection. The slightly increased risk of atopic disorders in breast-fed infants may be a consequence of a reduced incidence of gastrointestinal infection or more hygienic childcare.

Environmental Factors

Both indoor and outdoor pollutants have been put forward as possible contributory factors to the increase in asthma seen in recent decades. Many members of the general public hold the belief that air pollution, such as that caused by urban traffic levels, is responsible for the increase in the incidence and severity of asthma. However, overall air pollution in the United Kingdom has fallen substantially since the 1950s, with concentrations of sulphur dioxide, oxides of nitrogen and other pollutants all much lower now than in the days of the infamous London 'smogs'. Hence, an increase in air pollution seems an unlikely explanation for the increase in asthma (Seaton A et al., 1994). This conclusion is supported by the findings of the American six cities study (Ware JH et al., 1986). In this study, no association was found between the prevalence of asthma and exposure to particulates, nitrogen dioxide or sulphur dioxide. In another study, which compared schoolchildren in the heavily polluted city of Leipzig and the much less polluted city of Munich, the prevalence of asthma and airways hyper-reactivity did not differ significantly between children in the two cities (Von Mutius E et al., 1992). Numerous changes in the indoor environment, particularly those that increase the numbers of house dust mites (eg central heating, double glazing, fitted carpets), are more likely to be important.

Natural History

Significant advances have been made in our knowledge of the natural history of asthma but surprisingly little is known about the prognosis in children with wheezing and asthma (Martinez FD, 1997). This is largely because the follow-up of patients in many studies has been short-term and also because selected populations, not always representative of children with asthma, have been followed up. The most comprehensive study of asthma prognosis is the ongoing clinical follow-up of wheezy children identified by a population survey of seven year olds in Melbourne, Australia, in 1964 (Williams H, 1969). As this group were followed up into adult life (Martin AJ et al., 1980; Kelly WJW et al., 1987), it became apparent that some children who had apparently grown out of their asthma experienced a relapse, whereas others, who had been symptomatic, remitted. This is an important area for future study because if the current prevalence rates of asthma in children persist into older age, this will have major implications for health services.

A similar pattern of remission and relapse was also seen in the British 1958 cohort study (Strachan DP et al., 1988). In this study, only 2% of children who had wheezed up to the age of seven years were reported to have had attacks of asthma or wheezy bronchitis in the past year at all follow-ups (ages 7, 11, 16 and 23). Most of the children who had no attacks of asthma or wheezy bronchitis at age seven remained free of illness at each subsequent follow-up. Thus, short-term prognostic studies of asthma give an incomplete picture of the natural history of the condition.

1. Consultation rates
Consultation rates per 10,000 patients per year

Age group	Year of survey		
	1971-72	*1981-82*	*1991-92*
0-4	24.9	71.3	204.5
5-14	43.3	72.9	148.6
15-24	24.3	38.3	74.6
25-44	27.3	31.9	58.7

2. Patients consulting
Percentage of patients consulting in 1 year

Age group	Year of survey		
	1971-72	*1981-82*	*1991-92*
0-4	1.1	2.6	8.6
5-14	1.4	2.9	7.7
15-24	0.8	1.7	4.4
25-44	0.8	1.2	3.0

Table 3.8 Consultation rates for asthma per 10,000 patients per year with general practitioners and percentage of patients consulting their general practitioner for asthma in one year in 1971-82, 1981-82 and 1991-92

Source: Based on information found in the following surveys: 1971-72, 1981-82 and 1991-92 National Morbidity Surveys.

GENERAL PRACTICE WORKLOAD

Workload in general practice from asthma has increased considerably in recent decades with large increases seen in both the percentages of patients consulting for asthma and in consultation rates (see Table 3.8).

The percentage of under five year olds consulting for asthma in one year, increased from 1.1% in 1971-72 to 8.6% in 1991-92. During the same period consultation rates for asthma in this age group increased from 25 per 1,000 to 205 per 1,000; an eight-fold increase. In part, the increases in both number of patients and workload is a result of the improvements seen in general practice over the last 30 years. General practitioners are now much better at identifying and treating chronic diseases such as asthma and also at record keeping. However, some of the increase in the workload from asthma, especially among children, will have been a consequence of the increase in the prevalence and severity of asthma that has occurred over the same period of time.

PRESCRIBING IN GENERAL PRACTICE

Information on prescribing for asthma comes from two main sources: PACT and computerised medical records. PACT (Prescribing Analyses and CosTs) is derived from general practitioners' prescriptions and provides information on the quantity and cost of prescribing in general practice (Majeed A et al., 1997). Unfortunately, PACT does not include any demographic information, and so cannot be used to calculate prescribing rates for specific age groups. PACT also does not contain the indication for the drug prescribed, making it difficult to examine prescribing for specific diagnoses. For example, anti-asthmatic medication such as inhaled steroids and bronchodilators are often prescribed for patients with chronic airways disease. From PACT, we can obtain the total number of prescriptions issued but cannot determine how much of the prescribing was for asthma and how much for chronic airways disease.

In England, the total number of prescriptions of drugs used in the treatment of asthma increased by 27% between 1991 and 1996, with prescriptions for inhaled corticosteroids increasing at a faster rate than those for inhaled bronchodilators (see Figure 3.1).

Prescriptions for bronchodilators increased by 20% from about 15.5 million items in 1991 to 18.5 million items in 1996. During the same period, prescriptions of steroids increased by 74% from 6.3 to 10.9 million items. Prescriptions of antimuscarinic bronchodilators also increased between 1991 and 1996, but prescriptions of theophylline and cromoglycate fell. Trends in the cost of drugs used for the treatment of asthma show a similar trend, with the cost of corticosteroids increasing by 114% between 1991 and 1996 (see Figure 3.2).

DATA FROM GENERAL PRACTICE CONSULTATIONS

The General Practice Research Database (GPRD) collates information on prescribing and consultations from 400 practices, with a combined list size of about three million patients. All use the VAMP computer system. The information is collected for each patient and so it is feasible to carry out analyses that are not possible using PACT data.

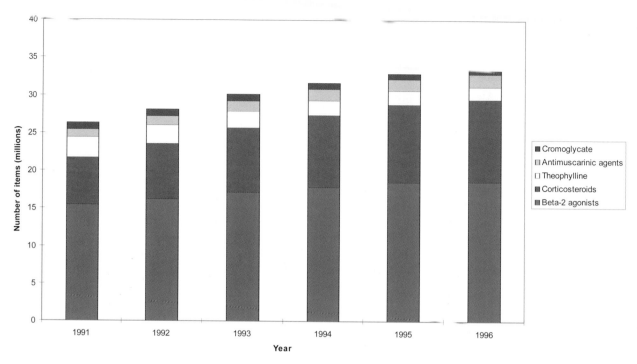

Figure 3.1 Annual number of items of drugs prescribed for the treatment of asthma in England, 1991-96

Source: Based on information provided by the Department of Health.

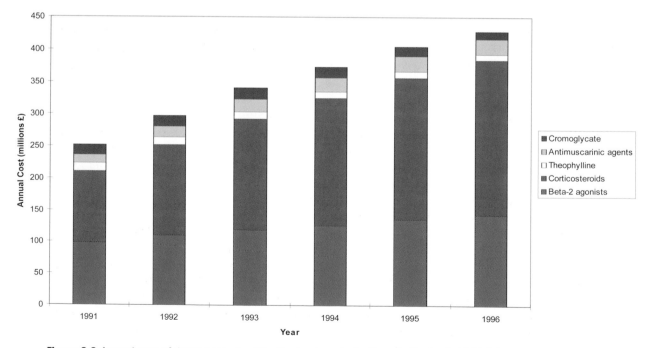

Figure 3.2 Annual cost of drugs prescribed for the treatment of asthma in England, 1991-96

Source: Based on information provided by the Department of Health.

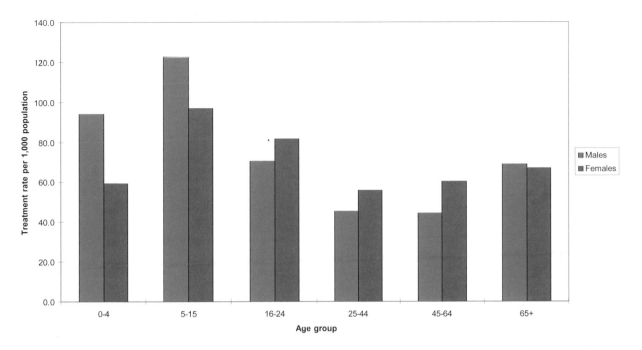

Figure 3.3 Number of people per 1,000 population receiving treatment for asthma in England and Wales in 1996

Source: Based on information provided by the Office for National Statistics.

The most recent analysis from GPRD was published in 1999, based on prescribing data for 1994 to 1996 (Majeed, 1999). Data from the GPRD show that the proportion of people in England and Wales who were being treated for asthma in 1996 was highest in the 5 to 15 year old age group. A higher proportion of boys than girls were being treated for asthma but among young adults the opposite pattern was seen, with more women than men receiving treatment. Among people aged 65 years and over, a higher proportion of men than women received treatment for asthma (see Figure 3.3). Data from the GPRD also show that about 72% of patients with asthma were prescribed inhaled steriods in 1996.

INTER-PRACTICE VARIATION

Several researchers have examined the management of asthma in general practice by examining the variation in measures such as prescribing and admissions. Prescribing and admission rates for asthma were examined in 124 practices in East London (Griffiths C et al., 1997). Wide varia-

tions in hospital admission rates (annual mean admission rate in 5 to 64 year olds 0.9 per 1,000, range 0 to 3.6 per 1,000) was found and in the ratio of inhaled steroids to inhaled bronchodilators (mean ratio 0.34, range 0.09 to 0.63). Similar variations were found in a study of 99 practices in North Staffordshire (Shelley M et al., 1996). The explanations for such large variations in the management of asthma in general practice remain unclear and further work trying to understand their causes will be an important area for future research.

HOSPITAL ADMISSIONS

The total number of hospital admissions for asthma (in England and Wales) increased massively during the 1970s and 1980s. By the mid 1980s admissions were about 80,000 per year compared to under 20,000 per year in the early 1960s. More recent data from the 1990s show that the number of admissions have stabilised at around 100,000 per year, with children now accounting for about half of all of these.

The increase in asthma admissions might have arisen for a number of reasons, including changes in any of the following:

- prevalence of asthma
- severity of disease
- behaviour of patients (or their parents) during attacks of asthma
- more patients attending and being admitted from Accident and Emergency departments
- medical care factors, affecting the threshold of admission or the likelihood of re-admission
- changes in hospital information systems and in the coding of diseases

The largest increases in admission rates occurred in children. In England and Wales, annual admission rates in 0 to 4 year olds increased from 4 per 10,000 in 1962 to nearly 80 per 10,000 by 1985. The current admission rate for asthma in this group is about 90 per 10,000. Rates also increased nearly six-fold in 5 to 9 year olds to 40 per 10,000 by the mid 1980s. More recently these figures have decreased to 30 per 10,000 per year. Rates in 10 to 14 year olds have increased more slowly and now stand at about 22 per 10,000 per year.

The increases in admission rates in children cannot be explained completely by an increase in re-admissions, diagnostic transfer from related categories such as bronchiolitis, or changes in the threshold for admission (Anderson HR et al., 1989). A variety of medical care factors have been suggested as the cause of the increase, including more self-referral to Accident and Emergency departments during acute attacks, and an increase in referrals of children with acute asthma to hospital by general practitioners.

MORTALITY

Only a minute proportion of episodes of asthma result in death. For the individual general practitioner, the death of a patient from an acute asthmatic attack will be a rare event – perhaps only once in a career. Nevertheless, there were more than 1,300 deaths from asthma in England and Wales in 1996. Although most of these occurred in people aged 65 years and over, there were 459 deaths in people aged under 65 years, many of

which may have been preventable, and most of which will have had preventable factors. Deaths from asthma in children are very rare events with just 20 deaths in 0 to 14 year olds in England and Wales in 1996. Examination of the annual number of deaths since 1958 shows that there were two peaks in deaths, in the mid 1960s and in the late 1980s (see Figure 3.4).

The first peak in the 1960s was ascribed initially to the use of inhaled isoprenaline, a short-acting inhaled bronchodilator released in the 1960s, which may have cardiotoxic effects if administered during episodes of hypoxia. Later, analysis suggested that although there was an undoubted association between the inhaler and deaths, there may have been a failure to appreciate the severity of asthma and use of other treatments. A second peak in asthma deaths occurred in the late 1980s and by 1988 there were over 2,000 deaths from asthma in England and Wales. Since 1988, the number of deaths has fallen steadily (see Figure 3.5).

Death rates have fallen in all age groups, with the largest falls observed in older people. There will be a number of reasons for this fall, particularly the considerable advances in general practice based management of the condition over the past ten years.

A recent analysis of social class differences in death rates from asthma, carried out by the Office for National Statistics, found that standardised mortality ratios for asthma were over four times higher in men from social class five than in men from social class one (Drever F et al., 1997). This outcome (see Figure 3.6) probably reflects a combination of factors: poor compliance with treatment, inadequate access to health services, and a higher prevalence of behaviours that have an adverse effect on health (such as smoking). The very small number of deaths from asthma in children, make it difficult to interpret social class differences in death rates in this group.

CONCLUSIONS

The epidemiology of asthma has changed significantly in recent decades with the prevalence of asthma, and other atopic disorders, increasing

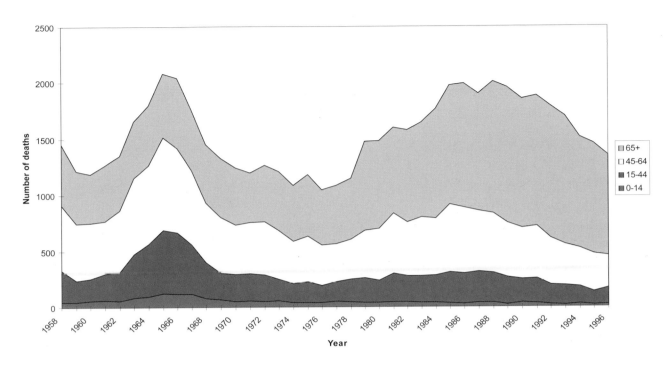

Figure 3.4 Annual number of deaths from asthma in England and Wales, 1958-96

Source: Based on information provided by the Office for National Statistics.

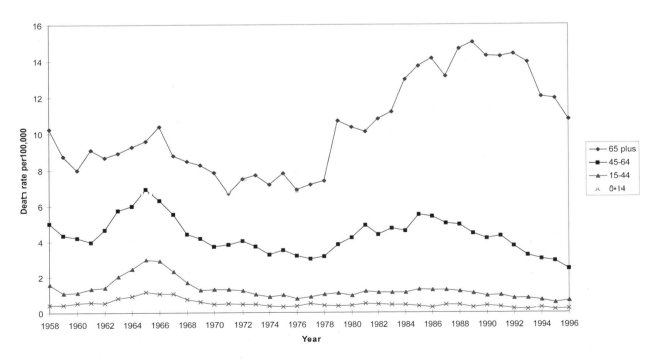

Figure 3.5 Annual death rates per 100,000 from asthma in England and Wales, 1958-96

Source: Based on information provided by the Office for National Statistics.

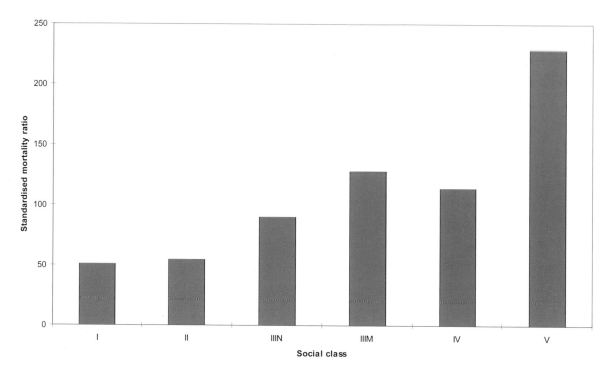

Figure 3.6 Standardised mortality ratios for asthma by social class in men aged 20-64, 1991-93

Source: Based on information provided by the Office for National Statistics.

markedly. The explanation for the increase in the prevalence is not entirely clear but air pollution seems unlikely to be the cause. Changes in the indoor environment, and in the exposure to allergens and infectious disease during early life, seem more likely to be responsible. The increase in prevalence, combined with better management of asthma in primary care, has resulted in a large increase in consultation rates for asthma, especially among children. Other measures of the utilisation of health services, such as admission and prescribing rates, have also increased in recent decades. Despite the increase in the prevalence of asthma, death rates from asthma peaked in the late 1980s and have fallen steadily since that time, probably reflecting better management of asthma in both primary and secondary care.

4

Diagnosis and Investigations

Introduction

Primary care physicians and nurses face various issues in determining a provisional diagnosis of asthma. Following this, patients need to be reassessed:

- in order to reaffirm the diagnosis (particularly in the case of young children)
- to determine their level of asthma control
- in older patients, to establish whether the diagnosis is chronic obstructive pulmonary disease (COPD), asthma or a combination of the two

In this chapter, the common and uncommon presenting symptoms at all ages are described and the confirmation of the diagnosis and differentiation from COPD is discussed. In order to improve and encourage early, accurate diagnosis of asthma the focus will be on those patients who present in more unusual ways.

Why the label 'Asthma'?

In the past many health professionals were reluctant to label patients with a diagnosis of asthma. This situation now seems to have reversed and there is a need to scrutinise the accuracy of diagnosis, and be aware of the possibility of over diagnosis! Health professionals should make an objective assessment of the patient. After confirming the diagnosis, the health professional should enter the term asthma in the patient's medical record and ensure that the patient and their family are made fully aware of the nature of the illness. These two steps alone will assist clinical management and result in a greater likelihood of adjusting asthma medication rather than adding antibiotics when patients consult with uncontrolled asthma. Furthermore, the parents of a distressed asthmatic child may be more likely to get rapid assistance when telephoning the doctor or ambulance service for urgent help than, for example, in the case of a report of 'chestiness'. Use of the term 'asthma' by patients is more likely to result in an urgent appointment with the general practitioner and is helpful for the ambulance service in their triage system for prioritising calls. Encouraging self-help for patients and health promotion is very important. Those patients who have not been given a specific diagnosis are less able to inform or help themselves in their struggle against asthma.

In general, the reasons for using the term 'asthma' outweigh the main reason against, ie a fear of provoking anxiety amongst parents and patients. Wheezy infants in the first year of life are perhaps the only exception to this rule. The pathophysiological definition of asthma in very young children is unclear. Therefore, it is suggested that the terms 'wheezing illness' or 'infantile asthma' are used in these infants (The British Thoracic Society et al., 1997) and that the diagnosis should be reconsidered at regular intervals.

In the 1980s, underdiagnosis was a major problem. Since Speight and others (Tudor Hart, 1986; Heeijne den Bak, 1986; Toop, 1985; Levy and Bell, 1984; Speight, 1978; Speight et al., 1983) highlighted the appalling level of underdiagnosis and management, those working in primary care have excelled themselves in their approach to diagnosis and management. The national levels of diagnosis have increased to around 15% in the case of children and approaching 7% in adults. However, although asthma diagnosis has improved in primary care, there is concern that many children may be inappropriately diagnosed without due consideration of the history and objective measurements of pulmonary function. An incorrect diagnosis of asthma may result in inappropriate increased levels of treatment when symptoms remain unresolved. Therefore it is essential that the diagnosis and status (eg controlled current asthma, uncontrolled current asthma, in remission) are reviewed from time to time.

The principles discussed in this chapter are relevant to the continued assessment of uncontrolled asthma as well as the initial diagnosis. Because of the long and unpredictable natural history of the condition, diagnostic skills are required for exacerbations, and sometimes for relapse after years of remission.

CHILDREN

1. Symptoms

At least 1 in 7 children in the United Kingdom have asthma. When children consult with respiratory symptoms and have a family history of atopy, eczema or asthma, or a personal history of the first two, this points towards a possible diagnosis of asthma. Symptoms are often precipitated by upper respiratory tract infections, are usually worse at night and are likely to be triggered by exercise. Presentation tends to follow two patterns: acute wheezy episodes (induced by a variety of precipitating factors) and recurrent day to day symptoms (Silverman and Wilson, 1995). The physical examination is often normal, despite a history of pronounced nocturnal symptoms, and hence the diagnosis is often missed. Specific questions should be asked in order to identify other clues to assist in the diagnosis of asthma (see Table 4.1).

According to some textbooks, 'wheezing' is the diagnostic symptom of asthma in children. However, cough rather than wheeze is the commonest presenting symptom of children with asthma in general practice. A particular pattern of this disease - 'cough variant asthma' - was first mentioned in 1975 by McFadden, who described 21 patients with this problem. These children suffered from exertional dyspnoea or cough as their dominant symptom and he concluded that asthma should be considered in similar cases. It seems this is a relatively common form of asthma, often not recognised by health professionals. The clue to diagnosis lies in the recurrent nature of the cough, which may be spontaneous or in response to trigger factors.

A common misconception held by doctors is that it is 'normal' for children to consult frequently with respiratory symptoms. This may result in inappropriate diagnosis of bronchitis or 'chestiness', and treatment of infection rather

Common	Uncommon
Family history:	Prodromal itching
asthma	Vomiting
eczema	Chest pain
allergies	
atopy	
parents who smoke	
Symptoms precipitated by:	
infections	
excitement	
laughter	
cold weather	
dust	
smoke	
pollen	
animals	
Cough:	
night	
recurrent	
dry/productive	
persists for long time	
Wheeze	
Disturbed nights	
Exercise intolerance	

Table 4.1 Clues to the diagnosis of asthma in childhood

than asthma. In fact studies have shown that children without asthma do not consult so frequently for respiratory symptoms. Therefore any child attending the surgery more than three times in any year with respiratory symptoms (cough, wheeze or shortness of breath), should be considered asthmatic until proved otherwise (Levy, 1986; Levy et al., 1985; Levy and Bell, 1984).

2. Clues to diagnosis by using medical records

In the UK, the National Health Service general practice records are important tools in the diagnosis of childhood asthma when patients present with respiratory symptoms. These records are complete from birth onwards and are sent to each new doctor with whom the patient registers; this facilitates diagnosis where there have been numerous previous respiratory consultations (Levy, 1986; Levy et al., 1985; Levy and Bell, 1984).

Two illustrative case histories (see Tables 4.2 and 4.3), first published in *Asthma in Practice* (Levy and Hilton, 1987), show the respiratory consultations of children.

Date	Symptom	Treatment
09.12.81	Coughing	Antibiotic
29.12.81	Coughing (still)	Antibiotic
04.01.82	Coughing (still) diagnosis pertussis	
11.01.82	Coughing	
01.02.82	Coughing – not sleeping	Phenergan
08.02.82	Coughing – not sleeping	
	Chest X-ray	
22.02.82	Coughing – hospital referral	
	Is this asthma?	
21.09.82	Coughing	Antitussive/antibiotic
05.10.82	Coughing (still)	
12.11.82	Coughing	Antibiotic
07.02.83	Coughing	Antibiotic
14.02.83	Coughing (still) – diarrhoea	Stop Px
28.02.83	Coughing/wheezing	Bronchodilator
14.03.83	Coughing (still)	Continue bronchodilator
28.03.83	No cough	**Asthma diagnosed**

Table 4.2 Case history illustrating respiratory consultations in a male patient, born 18 September 1981

Source: Levy M and Hilton SR (1987) Asthma in Practice. London, RCGP.

Date	Symptom	Treatment
01.08.78	Coughing	Phenobarbitone
23.11.79	Coughing	Antitussive
21.05.80	Coughing	Antitussive
04.11.80	Coughing	Antitussive/antibiotic
18.11.80	Coughing (still)	Antitussive
20.02.81	Coughing (for months)	
	Chest X-ray	
02.11.81	Coughing	Antibiotic
30.11.81	Coughing	Antitussive
04.02.82	Coughing, not sleeping	Antitussive
09.03.82	Coughing	Antitussive
18.03.82	Coughing	Antitussive/antibiotic
29.06.82	Coughing	Antitussive
26.08.82	Coughing	Antitussive
10.11.83	Coughing	Antitussive
18.11.83	Coughing (still)	Antitussive
12.12.83	Coughing (still)	Antibiotic
23.12.83	Follow-up – some improvement	
06.01.84	Coughing (still)	Multivitamin mixture
30.01.84	Coughing – peak flow rate = 250 L/M	
	= normal for height. Asked child to do a	
	peak flow chart over the next week	
03.02.84	Peak flow chart reading varied from	
	200 L/M to 240 L/M = 20% variation:	
	Diagnosis asthma. Prescribed terbutaline via spacer inhaler	
09.04.84	Review appointment: doing well PFR 250 L/M	

Table 4.3 Case history illustrating respiratory consultations in a female patient, born 29 October 1975

Source: Levy M and Hilton SR (1987) Asthma in Practice. London, RCGP.

Case history 1

For the purpose of this discussion, this child's history has been summarised to show his consultations for respiratory problems; that is, cough, wheeze, shortness of breath and difficulty in sleeping (see Table 4.2). It is clear that although he first presented with these symptoms at the age of three months, his asthma was not diagnosed until he was two and a half years old, and after 15 consultations for respiratory symptoms. Note the entries which state 'still coughing' and 'not sleeping' and also the many repeat consultations despite therapy with antitussives and antibiotics.

Case history 2

Table 4.3 tells a similar story, but in this case a child with asthma was left undiagnosed for nearly six years, after 20 consultations for respiratory symptoms. Note the clues to the diagnosis in the form of the entries 'still coughing', 'coughing for months' and 'not sleeping'. Also note the frequent repeat consultations and the fact that this child never consulted with the symptom of wheeze.

Although these case histories are relatively old, it is still not uncommon to find this pattern of delayed diagnosis. The histories of these two children clearly demonstrate the clues to the diagnosis, namely the words 'cough', 'still coughing', 'coughing for months' and 'wheezing'.

In a study of 52 asthmatic children (Levy and Bell, 1984), one third had the presenting symptom of difficulty in sleeping - shown clearly in the two case histories. The ratio of consultations was far higher for cough than wheeze. In addition, the prescriptions for these respiratory consultations were mainly for antitussives and antibiotics. A further study comparing the number of respiratory consultations in 52 diagnosed asthmatics with those of 69 normal children, confirmed that the asthmatics consulted significantly more frequently and lends support to the assertion that asthma should be considered in frequent respiratory attenders (Levy et al., 1985) A more recent follow-up study of 106 children with 'chronic cough' for two years in primary care found that 71 had asthma (Spelman, 1991).

Complete primary care records (such as those in the UK) are useful in screening for asthma. Toop (1985) was able to show that the medical records could be reliably screened for asthma. He scored the records of 225 children by allocating points for the following words and phrases: 'atopic eczema', 'nocturnal cough', 'persistent cough', 'still coughing', 'wheezing' or 'bronchodilator drug prescriptions'. There was a strong relationship between the screening score and post-exercise bronchoconstriction, thus confirming the value of suspecting asthma in those patients with recurrent respiratory symptoms. Den Bak was later able to double the diagnosed prevalence of asthmatic children in his practice from 7% to 15%. He screened the records for keywords ('asthma', 'wheeze', 'bronchitis', 'wheezy bronchitis', recurrent 'chest infection', 'nocturnal cough', 'eczema/atopy', 'hay fever', 'Ventolin', 'Bricanyl' and other bronchodilators) and subsequently recalled patients for assessment (Heeijne den Bak, 1986).

Bryce and colleagues targeted 3,373 children (aged 1 to 15 years) for clinical review. The children were identified by an audit facilitator who searched for case record entries suggestive of asthma. The twelve participating general practices found significant increases in attendance, diagnoses of asthma and confirmation of the diagnoses compared with the control group (Bryce et al., 1995).

Most children with asthma, therefore, can be diagnosed by careful history and scrutiny of the records of those consulting with multiple recurrent respiratory symptoms. The practice nurse (see Chapter 9) or receptionist could be encouraged to screen the records of new patients for keywords as described above. The common UK practice of routinely sorting new patients' records chronologically provides an opportunity for screening out those previously undiagnosed asthmatics. The subject of diagnosis of asthma lends itself very well to medical audit and research (see Chapter 10).

Toop (1985)	Den Bak (Heeijne den Bak, 1986)

All children born in 1 year (1977)
Identified using age-sex register
Records were scrutinised
Records were scored – 1 point for each entry of:
    Atopic eczema (after age 6 months)
    Nocturnal asthma
    Persisting cough (over 1 week,
    'still coughing', 'cough persists')
    Wheezing
    Bronchodilator used
Children performed exercise tests
	All children under 16 years
	
	Records were scrutinised
	The following keywords were identified in the notes:
	    Asthma
	    Wheeze
	    Bronchitis
	    Recurrent chest infection
	    Nocturnal cough
	    Eczema/atopy/hayfever
	    Ventolin/bricanyl
	
	All children with 1 keyword were
	interviewed and examined
	A group of children with no keyword were
	sent a questionnaire and children with
	history of any of the above keywords
	were recalled for examination

Conclusions: 1) Medical record scrutiny is helpful in identifying possible asthmatic children 2) Presentation of asthma varies: the repeated presence of any of the above features justifies a trial of asthma therapy; the more features present in any one child the more likely the child has asthma	Conclusions: 1) Keywords identified in records and by questionnaire were helpful in identifying children with asthma 2) Examination of children with positive keywords was helpful in establishing who required more treatment

Table 4.4 Asthma diagnosis screening – two examples of method

3. Delayed diagnosis

Reasons for the delay in diagnosis relate mostly to weaknesses in the organisation of care in general practice (Levy, 1986). The time pressure during consultations may contribute to inadequate history taking. The lack of continuity of care resulting from multiple consultations with different doctors occurs mainly in group practices but includes sole practitioners who need locum cover during periods of absence. Change of doctor, often with the unacceptable time taken to transfer past medical records (from previous doctor to health authority/health board to new doctor), may also delay the diagnosis. However, a routine interview (or written questionnaire) detailing the past medical history of new patients should help to overcome this problem. Tudor Hart (1986) suggested that diagnostic denial by doctors was of relevance; he found a marked delay in the diagnosis of asthma in his practice with 30% of children taking more than 15 consultations before diagnosis. Other authors concluded that the use of the term 'bronchitis' to denote recurrent respiratory problems in children detracted from the diagnosis of asthma (Jones and Sykes, 1990).

More recent evidence suggests that asthma is being diagnosed earlier by members of the primary care team (Levy et al., 1996; Levy et al., 1998; Levy 1994; Charlton et al., 1991). In 1993, two cohort studies of children with asthma in 125 practices in North London, showed that the mean age of diagnosis of asthma reduced from 6.7 years (95% ci 6.3 to 7.1) to 3.4 years (95% ci 3.2 to 3.7) in those born in 1982 and 1987 respectively (Levy and Bland, 1993). In 1996, another study of 466 practices in the UK also demonstrated a reduction in the age at diagnosis of children born in 1987 compared to a group born in 1988. This was part of a one-year randomised study to investigate the effect of training nurses in asthma management on the change in overall care delivered by their practices. The reduction in age diagnosed was statistically significant in the active group, where practice

	Born 1987	**Born 1988**
	Age diagnosed (95% ci)	Age diagnosed (95% ci)
Active group	3.95 (3.87 - 4.01)* n=2022	3.75 (3.63 - 3.85)* n=944
Control group	4.03 (3.96 - 4.1) n=2279	3.92 (3.83 - 4) n=1399

* statistically significant differences

Table 4.5 Demonstrating a reduction in the age of asthma diagnosis ie reduction in the delay in diagnosing children with asthma (Levy et al., 1998)

nurses were following up a selected group of patients within their practice. These data are shown in Table 4.5 (Levy et al., 1998).

While this provides welcome evidence that asthma is being diagnosed earlier in primary care, further research to determine the accuracy of diagnoses is desirable. It is difficult to be sure in the case of young children, whether asthma has been correctly diagnosed, hence the need for regular re-evaluation. It is noteworthy that over 60% of the children in the study above were prescribed inhaled steroids at that time. Accurate diagnosis is essential in order to ensure appropriate prescription of this therapy.

4. Atypical presentations of childhood asthma

Some children present with more unusual symptoms. In a review of 'variant forms of asthma' Miser (Miser, 1987) described one of his patients, a 13-year-old girl who had a three-year history of intermittent chest pain. The child's pain was located substernally, lasted 30 seconds, and was sometimes associated with dyspnoea, but she never wheezed. She was extensively investigated and, because of a slightly low peak flow reading, was prescribed cromoglycate and a bronchodilator. After four months of treatment, the pain had resolved and all other symptoms had disappeared. Miser cites other similar examples in his review. Chest pain should therefore be considered as a presenting feature of asthma, especially in children.

Severe recurrent vomiting has been described as another variant presenting symptom of asthma.

Schreier and colleagues first described five children aged 11 months to 9 years with this uncommon form of asthma. The same authors later described another three cases, two children aged 33 months and five years, and a 41-year-old man (Schreier et al., 1984 and 1987). These patients usually had a past history of asthma, or a family or personal history of allergy and eczema. Previous similar episodes are an important clue to the diagnosis and patients may have been investigated to no avail by gastroenterologists. Episodes usually begin with mild to moderate cough which follows an upper respiratory infection, and this is followed by severe repeated vomiting which may contain only mucus, but which always does contain mucus. Wheeze is often present after the patient starts to recover from the episode. Children may become dehydrated rapidly and require urgent treatment with intravenous fluids, bronchodilators and steroids. The authors excluded whooping cough in those cases, and postulated neurologic crossconnections in the medullary cough and vomit centres as a possible mechanism for this form of asthma. We suspect that there are probably more children who present with these features, and can recollect acute asthmatics presenting with coughing who were difficult to manage where a diagnosis of asthma would have probably simplified therapy. In support of evidence of vomiting as a symptom of asthma Anderson et al (Anderson et al., 1987), in a national cohort of over 8,000 children, were able to relate periodic abdominal pain or vomiting attacks in children and future development of asthma.

Prodromal symptoms of asthma

A surprising case occurred when an 11-year-old boy presented with a 'tingly back' (Levy, 1985). On auscultation he had a wheezy chest and his peak flow rate was low. His records detailed 15 respiratory consultations over eight years and he gave a history of exercise-induced breathlessness. He was suffering from 'prodromal itching' which had been previously described in two prospective studies which found the prevalence of itching associated with asthma to be 41% (David et al., 1984) and 70% (Orr, 1979). This condition, as well as other prodromal symptoms of asthma attacks, are surprisingly consistent in particular children and can therefore be used to stimulate initiation of acute asthma treatment (Beer et al., 1987). The prodromal symptoms include: respiratory symptoms (cough, rhinorrhoea, and wheezing); behavioural changes (irritability, apathy, anxiety, and sleep disorders); gastrointestinal symptoms (abdominal pain and anorexia); fever; itching; skin eruptions and toothache. These are usually recognised by asthmatic children, often unknown to the parents (Beer et al., 1987).

ASTHMA IN ADULTS

1. Symptoms

Adult asthma presents typically with symptoms of cough, wheeze and chest tightness, and is usually easy to diagnose in these circumstances. However, adult asthma remains underdiagnosed and clinicians need to bear this diagnosis in mind whenever patients present with respiratory symptoms. Recurrent symptoms, particularly related to asthma triggers provide a clue to the diagnosis.

Differentiation of Chronic Obstructive Pulmonary Disease (COPD) from patients with asthma becomes increasingly important with advancing age, and may be very difficult. Sometimes the two conditions coexist; these people need to be identified in order to institute appropriate management.

COPD is defined as a chronic, slowly progressive disorder characterised by airways obstruction ($FEV_1 < 80\%$ predicted and FEV_1 / FVC ratio $< 70\%$) which does not change markedly over several months. The impairment of lung function is largely fixed but may be partially reversible by bronchodilator (or other therapy). The term, COPD, encompasses a number of other terms including: chronic bronchitis, emphysema, chronic obstructive airways disease, chronic airflow limitation and some cases of chronic asthma (The COPD Guidelines Group of the Standards of Care Committee of the BTS, 1997).

Spirometry, rather than PEF, is appropriate in the diagnosis of COPD. Access to hospital lung function laboratories is variable and not all provide a service accessible to primary care physicians. However, advances in technological development have resulted in miniaturisation and a marked reduction in the cost of spirometers, improving their accessibility for general practitioners. A reversibility test to bronchodilators and corticosteroids is required in order to determine whether a patient would respond to therapy. An increase of 200ml and at least 15% from baseline of FEV_1 is indicative of this.

A study in Leeds comparing 201 people with asthma (diagnosed by general practitioners) with 113 diagnosed with chronic bronchitis, attempted to clarify whether the diagnosis could be made clinically and whether reversibility could be predicted clinically (Wardman et al., 1986). Their data are still relevant and helpful. While men and women were equally prevalent in the asthma group, there were twice as many men as women in the chronic bronchitis. Six symptoms were found to be useful in differentiating the two groups (see Table 4.6). There was considerable overlap in the two groups with respect to airflow reversibility. Sixty per cent of those with asthma and 22% of those with chronic bronchitis had a PEF reversibility of at least 15%. It is unclear whether patients with reversible airflow obstruction in combination with COPD have got true asthma. It seems sensible to treat these people with asthma medication. The current guidelines on COPD advise that we should first clearly demonstrate reversibility to bronchodilators and then to inhaled steroids (or oral steroids) and then treat if there is a positive response. The use of inhaled topical steroids should be limited to COPD patients who are proved to improve on this therapy.

Chronic bronchitis	Asthma (Wardman et al., 1986)
Chronic cough (with expectoration)	Hay fever
	Exercise-induced wheeze
Persisting symptoms	Episodic wheeze with Symptom-free periods
Onset over age 20	Onset of symptoms before the age of 20 years
History of smoking	All time nonsmokers

Table 4.6 Differentiating chronic obstructive pulmonary disease (COPD) from asthma

Source: Wardman et al., 1986. Published in the British Journal of Diseases. Reproduced with permission of WB Saunders Company Ltd.

2. Drug precipitants of adult-onset asthma

Side effects of beta-blocking agents such as propranolol, have long been known to precipitate airflow obstruction. Other drugs associated with asthma include aspirin and non-steroidal anti-inflammatory agents (such as ibuprofen) which may be dispensed as an oral or topical formulation. This is worrying because of the increasing availability of these drugs over the pharmacist's counter without prescription. The pharmaceutical industry and the high street pharmacists have a responsibility to inform the public of the dangers of these drugs for people with asthma. However, in our experience this does not always occur.

3. Occupational asthma

Occupationally induced asthma should be considered in any adults developing late onset asthma and where the symptoms seem associated with work periods. The diagnosis should be considered in those symptomatic patients who work in bakeries, paint, glue or the plastic industries. A two hourly peak flow diary is often required to confirm the diagnosis and ideally, patients suspected with this condition should be referred to a specialist with expertise in occupational asthma. Often, occupational asthma resolves with removal from exposure. This does not mean that these people should lose their jobs; arrangements should be made in discussion between the occupational physician and the employers. Compensation is available for certain categories of occupational asthma and relevant literature should be made available for patients.

Figure 4.1 shows the NAC leaflet on occupational asthma entitled 'Asthma at work'. There is a leaflet available from the Health and Safety Executive (HSE) entitled 'Preventing Asthma at Work: how to control respiratory Sensitisers'. The DSS pamphlet, Occupational Asthma NI 237, describes the situations where people may be entitled to disablement and other benefits.

4. Elderly patients

There are other ways in which asthma may present in elderly patients. There is a paucity of data in this regard and we suggest this subject for audit and research in primary care. A delay in

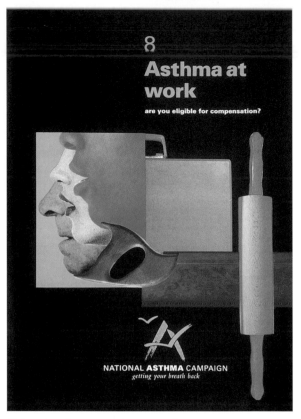

Figure 4.1 The National Asthma Campaign (NAC) produce many useful leaflets. This one 'Asthma at work' provides information on the aetiology of occupational asthma and aspects related to therapy and compensation

diagnosis ranging from 6 days to 4 years was described in a study of 13 elderly asthmatics (mean age 79 years) in whom the diagnosis was missed initially (Allen, 1988). The diagnoses were chronic obstructive airways disease in five, heart failure in three, bronchitis in one, and no diagnosis in the others. According to Allen, these patients may present with one of the so called 'geriatric giants' (falls, declining mobility, incontinence, confusion and social breakdown). A random survey of 1 in 8 people aged 70 and over, in South Wales in 1979, found a current prevalence of asthma in 5.1% of men and 1.8% in the women (Burr et al., 1979). In the patients with 'mild asthma' (diagnosed on typical histories and relief from bronchodilators) these figures are 7.9% for men and 5.7% for women. Asthma is therefore being misdiagnosed in many elderly patients and this results in inappropriate therapy.

There are probably many patients who have chronic bronchitis with a reversible element of their airflow obstruction and who would therefore benefit from therapy. As Burr and colleagues (1979) point out, sputum production is common in asthmatics and therefore chronic asthmatics may be incorrectly diagnosed as 'bronchitics'.

As in the case of children, chest pain may be a presenting symptom of asthma in adults.

5. Non-respiratory symptoms

Frequent non-respiratory symptoms of acute asthma were described in an audit of 30 consecutive adult asthmatic patients (Shneerson, 1986). The symptoms divided into those preceding acute attacks and those occurring mainly during attacks. Tiredness, sleepiness and depression preceded asthma attacks in 12 of the 30 patients. Nose and throat symptoms occurred before 66% of attacks; these included blocked, itching or runny nose, sneezing and tickle in the throat. Thirst, skin itching or flushing preceded a quarter of attacks. Other symptoms which occurred mainly during attacks include: palpitations, sweating or dizziness in a third of patients; dry mouth, thirst in some; and tiredness, sleepiness, depression, aches and pains, and increased urinary frequency in others.

CONFIRMING THE DIAGNOSIS

Use of the peak flow meter

Having suspected asthma from the history, the diagnosis can be confirmed in the surgery or clinic in most cases (see Figure 4.2). If the peak expiratory flow (PEF) reading is lower than expected (according to the normogram), give the patient a few puffs of beta-2 agonist bronchodilator (salbutamol or terbutaline), ask him/her to sit in the waiting room while other patients are seen, and then retest the PEF after 15 minutes. Calculate the PEF variation as described in Table 4.7. A variation exceeding 15% confirms significant reversible airway obstruction and therefore, asthma. A false negative result may occur if the dose of beta-2 agonist bronchodilator is not properly administered. Inhaler devices are difficult to use; therefore when doing a reversibility test it would be wise to use one of the large spacer

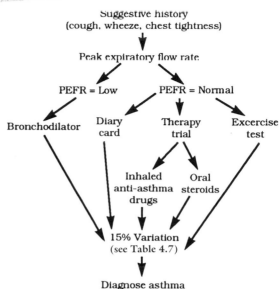

Figure 4.2 Confirmation of the diagnoses of asthma

Source: modified from Levy M (1987). Reproduced with permission.

devices (Volumatic for salbutamol, Nebuhaler for terbutaline) or a nebuliser.

A common mistake in diagnosing asthma is the assumption that a single normal peak flow reading excludes the diagnosis. The peak flow chart in Figure 4.3a demonstrates how misleading single readings taken in the surgery may be. However, the variation seen in the complete diurnal chart (see Figure 4.3b) provides evidence for confirmation of the diagnosis.

Calculating variability of peak expiratory flow

$$\frac{\text{Highest reading} - \text{lowest reading}}{\text{Highest reading}} \times 100$$

The following readings have been obtained over a week by measuring them twice daily.

AM PM AM PM AM PM AM PM AM PM AM PM
340 350 350 400 320 350 360 400 310 320 300 390

$$\frac{400 - 310}{400} \times 100 = 22.5\%$$

This variability is above 15% and therefore this patient has evidence of reversible airflow obstruction confirming the diagnosis of asthma.

Table 4.7 Calculating peak expiratory flow variation

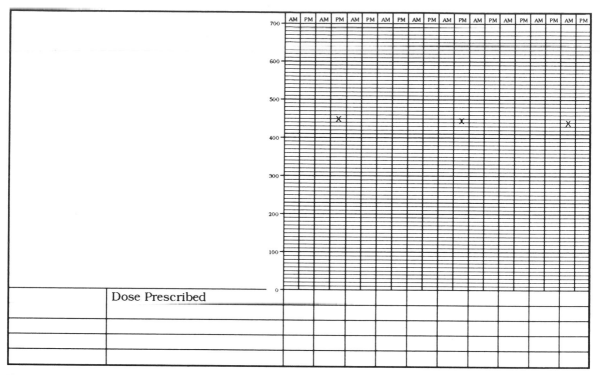

Figure 4.3a Three peak flow readings taken on different days

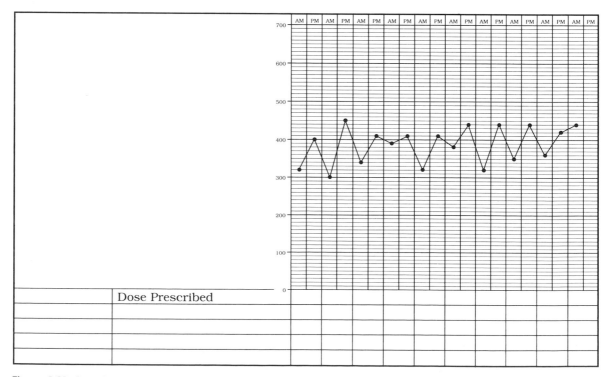

Figure 4.3b Complete diurnal chart for patient in Figure 4.3a

Because patients may take a few days to learn to use the meter properly, it is best to disregard the first few days' readings of a serial diary chart for diagnostic purposes. The standard peak expiratory flow normograms are unhelpful in determining whether the patient has airflow obstruction, because there is such a wide range of 'normal' readings. It is therefore important to utilise the variability of readings and not the absolute readings. The patient's peak expiratory flow may be appreciably below his or her usual best and yet be within the 'normal' range. Other patients are able to outperform the normal values. If the history is suggestive of asthma and the patient records a 'normal' peak flow rate, loan a peak flow meter to enable the patient to keep a twice daily record card for a few weeks. The variation may be calculated as described in Table 4.7 and if this is greater than 15% at any time, asthma should be diagnosed. If the symptoms are troublesome, a trial of anti-asthma therapy in addition may reduce the time taken to confirm the diagnosis by symptomatic as well as improved peak expiratory flow (increased levels and reduced variability). Occupational asthma may be confirmed in this way, although it is best to record two hourly PEF readings for this purpose.

Exercise testing

If the diagnosis is still in doubt and the history suggests asthma, then an exercise test may be of help. An exercise test should be performed only if rescue beta-2 agonist bronchodilators and resuscitation facilities are available. PEF or FEV_1 is measured before the test, and the patient is asked to run for 6 to 8 minutes. Another peak flow or FEV_1 reading is taken at the completion of the exercise and then again at five minute intervals for 15 to 20 minutes (Gibson, 1996). Calculate the variation, as in Table 4.7, and a figure exceeding 15% confirms the diagnosis.

Trial of steroids

A trial of oral or high dose inhaled steroid therapy (with intermittent rescue bronchodilators), in conjunction with PEF diary cards, is sometimes the only way of confirming the diagnosis. These drugs may need to be continued for three weeks before diagnosis can be confirmed or refuted. A trial of oral steroids is sometimes necessary; oral prednisolone is used for this purpose (30-60mg daily in adults; 0.5 to 2mg per kg/day in children. In children, usually not longer than one week and up to a maximum dose of 40mg per day). We suggest reviewing patients after a week in order to establish whether they are developing any side effects or if the diagnosis has been confirmed, in which case the dosages may be revised and oral steroids may be switched to an inhaled method of delivery.

SUMMARY

There are five good reasons for diagnosing asthma and using the term explicitly:

1. Asthma in undiagnosed asthmatics is not necessarily mild and patients may suffer considerably, missing a great deal of schooling or work.

2. The explicit use of the term asthma is more likely to lead to appropriate therapy.

3. Children do not necessarily grow out of their asthma and therefore it is best to get on with the job of advising parents and initiating treatment if appropriate.

4. Once diagnosed, the patient can be put in touch with the self-help organisations such as the National Asthma Campaign.

5. Chronic untreated asthma may result in physical disability such as chronic chest deformity, irreversible lung damage or even death. Psychological problems may result from a sense of invalidity, exclusion from sport, spoilt holidays, derision from school friends and inability to obtain work.

By maintaining a high index of suspicion, taking a careful detailed history, and recognising those patients presenting with respiratory symptoms, it may be possible to diagnose more asthma cases. In addition, it might be possible to reduce morbidity due to this disease by recognising uncontrolled asthma through applying the principles described above.

5

MANAGEMENT OF CHRONIC ASTHMA

INTRODUCTION

The focus of this chapter is the ongoing management of chronic asthma. Diagnosis has been discussed fully in Chapter 4; management of uncontrolled and acute severe asthma in Chapter 6; education in Chapter 7; and organisation of care (including clinics) in Chapter 9. Where relevant, some of these issues are discussed here.

The processes of the management of chronic asthma include: assessment and monitoring (with particular emphasis on determining whether patients' asthma is controlled); drug and device prescription; treatment modification; and education ensuring that patients understand how to treat their asthma as well as recognise when medical assistance is required.

We suggest a systematic way to achieve the best possible control of patients suffering from asthma. This approach may enable a busy clinician to determine rapidly whether:

- their patient has controlled or uncontrolled asthma
- immediate treatment is required
- the medication simply needs to be titrated up or down to the current level of control
- a specialist opinion is indicated

ASSESSMENT AND MONITORING

It is vital to appreciate that asthma is a chronic and labile condition that may go out of control at any time, in any patient. The principles underlying recognition of uncontrolled asthma are essentially the same as those used in the initial diagnosis (see Chapter 4). Patients and their families are important partners in the process of assessment and monitoring of asthma. By empowering patients to recognise and treat uncontrolled asthma and by ensuring availability of medical assistance when this fails, it should be possible to reduce morbidity and mortality due to asthma. This is more likely to happen if patients have been diagnosed early, given access to sources of self-help material, and followed up regularly by the doctor or practice nurse.

Assessment and monitoring by health professionals may take place in organised asthma clinics, or opportunistically during consultations for other medical problems. Many asthma patients will not attend for routine follow-up, making it necessary to assess their control when they consult for other problems. In fact, in many cases, asthma or allied conditions may even be partly accountable for the consultation. For example, patients presenting from the spring through to summer with 'colds' will be suffering from allergic rhinitis due to tree or grass pollens.

Given the nature of general practice it can be difficult, during a busy surgery, to focus upon a diagnosis unrelated to the main presenting complaint. A heightened awareness on the part of the clinician, of a patient's asthma status, may enable opportunistic monitoring of the condition to occur. A system of flagging the records (such as the RCGP coloured stickers) to identify these patients is helpful. Computerised records help in providing easy access to past medical history. If the possibility of uncontrolled asthma is kept in the forefront of the doctor's mind, it is less likely that the diagnosis will be missed. It is not uncommon for uncontrolled asthmatics to be misdiagnosed as suffering from chest infections. Indeed, these form a large proportion of patients referred inappropriately to outpatient departments.

While it is sometimes obvious when a patient presents with asthma symptoms, there are times

PATTERNS OF PRESENTATION OF CHILDHOOD ASTHMA

There are several clinical patterns of asthma in children in general practice. Different patterns may occur in the same child over a prolonged period as described below. Management decisions for these children need to be individually tailored based upon accepted national guidelines.

Persistent wheezing in infants
Onset of asthma certainly does occur under the age of one year but causes of wheezing other than asthma are more likely to occur in this age group than in older children. Wheezing during (and after) an attack of acute bronchiolitis is the commonest differential diagnosis

Persistent coughing in older children
Persistent coughing in older children, often without accompanying wheeze or obvious shortness of breath, is predominantly nocturnal and will probably be exacerbated by exercise or excitement. Closer questioning will often reveal a considerable curtailing of 'normal' activities

Asthma precipitated by viral URTIs
Asthma precipitated by viral upper respiratory tract infections, especially in younger children (that is, cough and wheeze only in association with an upper respiratory tract infection), is not often clinically severe. However, these children may miss time from school in the winter months and there may be low grade, undetected morbidity at other times.

Mild asthma with episodic symptoms
Children suffering from mild asthma with episodic symptoms tend to be older and possibly atopic. They may suffer an exacerbation as a result of exposure to high loads of allergen, such as mould or animal dander, or to an emotional upset or infection but seem to be symptom-free between episodes.

Continuous asthma
Continuous asthma is not necessarily severe enough to bring the child to the doctor with frequent exacerbations, but there are almost daily symptoms resulting from exercise or a change of atmosphere, and nocturnal symptoms, such as wheeze, but usually cough. This is the subgroup of children whose asthma is most likely to be underestimated by the practice and to be undertreated as a consequence.

Chronic severe asthma
Chronic severe asthma is uncommon in children. Their management is best supervised by a paediatrician but day-to-day advice and support from the family doctor is important.

Acute severe asthma
Acute severe asthma in childhood is discussed in Chapter 6.

when this is not so straightforward. Children with asthma tend to present in a number of ways due to their asthma. In the case of adults, there are sometimes difficulties in differentiating symptoms and signs resulting from various respiratory and cardiac conditions. Awareness of these patterns of presentation may be helpful when consulted by patients with respiratory symptoms.

It is the unpredictability and variability in presentation pattern which makes the management of asthma such a challenge and which means there is no room for complacency in dealing with the condition.

ASSESSING CONTROL OF ASTHMA
The aim of management of asthma is to abolish symptoms. While it is not always possible to control symptoms completely, it is important to determine whether the patient is in an unstable phase of asthma, and therefore liable to develop an attack. Therefore a health professional, when conducting a consultation for asthma monitoring, should aim to answer the following questions (see also box).

Has the patient currently (within the last month) had any symptoms of asthma (cough, wheeze and shortness of breath)?

Four questions the clinician should consider when consulted by patients with asthma:

1) Has the patient currently (within the last month) had any symptoms of asthma (cough, wheeze and shortness of breath)?
2) Does the patient obtain relief when using the rescue inhaler (ie the beta-2 agonist bronchodilator)?
3) Has the patient any evidence of reversible airflow obstruction?
4) Can the patient use the medication properly (ie the device and the timing of different medication, as well as the use of a self-management plan)?

This question will help to determine whether the patient is suffering from bronchial hyper-reactivity or 'twitchiness' of the airways. Many asthma patients may not be aware that they could function at a better level and often accept symptoms as a 'normal state of life'; in some cases even waking up coughing or wheezing almost every night. Many simply accept that they cannot take part in sport or even minimal exercise, and are loath to complain spontaneously about difficulty in breathing, sleeping, or problems related to mobility. The shift of emphasis in care towards prevention in medicine should be reflected in the doctor's approach to history taking. Patients should be questioned routinely about their symptoms and the effect of asthma upon their lifestyle.

Does the patient obtain relief when using the rescue inhaler (ie the beta-2 bronchodilator)?
A patient reporting that their symptoms are not relieved, or only improved for a short while by the reliever inhaler, has bronchial hyper-reactivity of significant proportion and is potentially at risk of developing a serious asthma attack. Immediate, aggressive treatment is required, probably including a short course of oral steroids (see Chapter 6).

Has the patient got evidence of reversible airflow obstruction?
This is defined as a 15% variation in PEF or FEV$_1$. Some patients' asthma may be uncontrolled

despite their perceived absence of symptoms and therefore objective measurements of lung function are required to identify and quantify the level of asthma control. Peak flow measurements before and after a beta-2 agonist bronchodilator can be carried in the surgery. A fifteen minute wait is necessary post bronchodilator, during which time other patients may be seen. Alternatively, patients may be asked to keep a diary chart for a week or two before attending; in this case it is helpful to ask the patient to annotate the chart with details of readings taken before and after medication or exercise.

Can the patient use the medication properly?
This question applies to the patients' ability to decide whether to initiate or increase certain

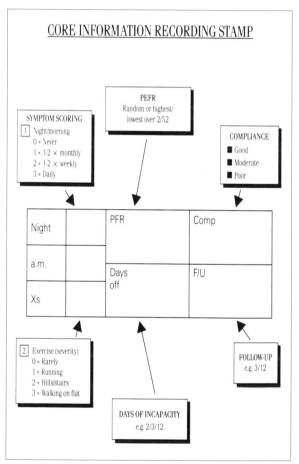

Figure 5.1 Core information recording stamp

Source: This rubber stamp for use in the patient's record is available from Action Asthma, Allen and Hanburys. We acknowledge our gratitude to the Tayside Asthma Group for kindly permitting us to reproduce this figure.

medications as well as their ability to self-administer these, ie the use of a self-management plan. For example, the patient should know when it would be appropriate to use reliever medication and when to increase existing anti-inflammatory inhaled steroids. How well does the patient use their inhaler device, and do they understand how to determine when this is empty?

The answers to these four questions place the clinician in a good position to decide how to adjust the patient's medication and whether additional resources are required.

A number of helpful tools may facilitate the monitoring process. The Tayside Asthma Group developed a rubber stamp (see Figures 5.1 and 5.2) which provides information on symptoms, PEF, compliance, exercise ability (or limitation) and days of incapacity. The National Asthma and Respiratory Training Centre (Warwick), sell a record card that fits neatly into the Lloyd George medical notes, used by most GPs in the UK. This card provides space for recording baseline information as well as an ongoing record of findings at each consultation (see Figure 5.3). These examples serve as an *aide memoire* as well as a means of recording accurate data for future audit.

Objective Monitoring of Lung Function in Asthma

Peak expiratory flow (PEF) is a reliable, convenient, cheap and a relatively simple method for monitoring asthma control. In addition this method offers patients and health professionals assistance in deciding whether, and by how much, to adjust medication. Self-monitoring with peak flow meters has been greatly helped by the availability of these devices on NHS prescription in the United Kingdom. Serial peak flow measurements provide an early objective measurement for asthma that is going out of control.

There is debate and uncertainty as to whether mild asthmatics should measure their peak flow regularly (see Chapter 7). It is our view that all moderate or severe asthmatic adults and older children (ie those old enough to use a meter properly) should have a peak flow meter. There are various situations in which the use of

peak flow measurements are particularly important – for example, when recovering from an attack and trying to decide whether to reduce steroid therapy, or when changing or stopping asthma therapy.

Patients should know what their normal or best achievable reading is. This is best determined during periods when feeling well as recorded in home diary charts. We believe that all severe asthmatics should check their readings regularly; while all patients on inhaled topical steroids should check their readings from time to time.

Patients should initiate regular daily peak flow readings (am and pm) whenever they suspect that symptoms are deteriorating and an attack may occur. PEF readings are usually lowest early in the morning (about 4am) and highest in the afternoon (about 4pm); readings should be recorded as close to these times as possible or practicable. Examples include: at the onset of an infection; when anticipating contact with known trigger factors; when moving to a new area; or when embarking on a major spring clean, or painting the house. It is easier for patients and/or parents to decide upon the need for therapeutic alterations if they are informed by readings from a peak flow diary. They can see at a glance whether the readings are 'normal' or if there is a wide variation.

Three early warning PEF signs of impending attacks are:

? decreasing levels

? increasing diurnal variation as seen by a widening gap between morning and evening readings

? early morning dips below the usual readings.

Calculation of PEF variability:

$$\frac{\text{Highest PEF} - \text{Lowest PEF}}{\text{Highest PEF}} \times 100$$

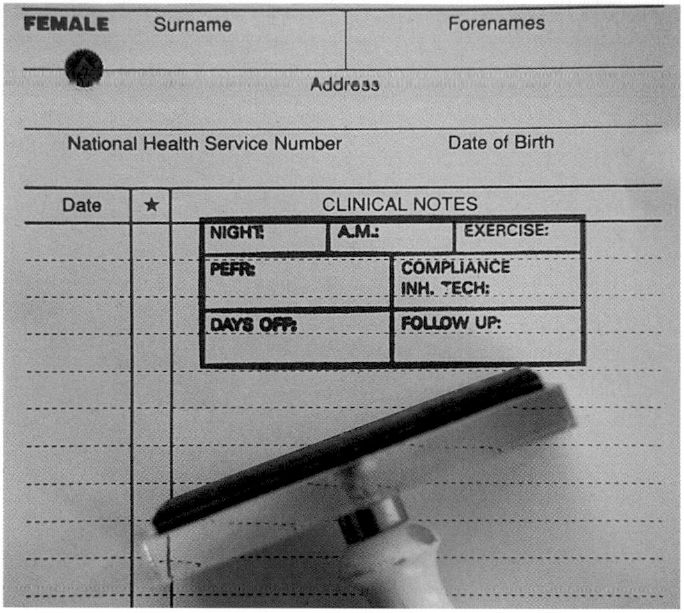

Figure 5.2 Photograph of the Tayside rubber stamp with box and imprint on records

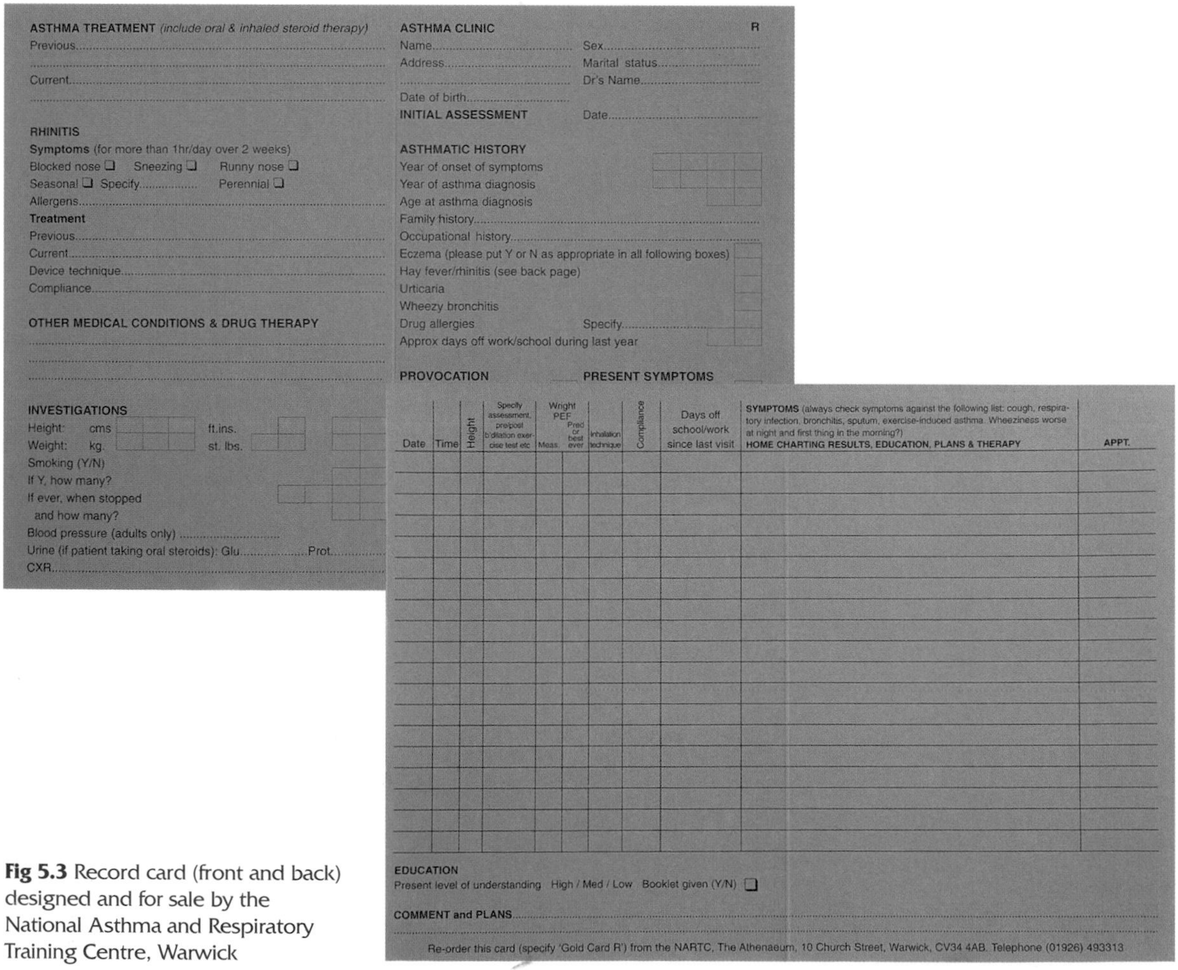

ASTHMA TREATMENT *(include oral & inhaled steroid therapy)*
Previous.......
Current.......

RHINITIS
Symptoms (for more than 1hr/day over 2 weeks)
Blocked nose ❑ Sneezing ❑ Runny nose ❑
Seasonal ❑ Specify........ Perennial ❑
Allergens.......
Treatment
Previous.......
Current.......
Device technique.......
Compliance.......

OTHER MEDICAL CONDITIONS & DRUG THERAPY

INVESTIGATIONS
Height: cms ft.ins.
Weight: kg. st. lbs.
Smoking (Y/N)
If Y, how many?
If ever, when stopped
and how many?
Blood pressure (adults only) ....
Urine (if patient taking oral steroids): Glu.......Prot.......
CXR.......

ASTHMA CLINIC R
Name....... Sex.......
Address....... Marital status.......
Dr's Name.......
Date of birth.......
INITIAL ASSESSMENT Date.......

ASTHMATIC HISTORY
Year of onset of symptoms
Year of asthma diagnosis
Age at asthma diagnosis
Family history.......
Occupational history.......
Eczema (please put Y or N as appropriate in all following boxes)
Hay fever/rhinitis (see back page)
Urticaria
Wheezy bronchitis
Drug allergies Specify.......
Approx days off work/school during last year

PROVOCATION PRESENT SYMPTOMS

Date	Time	Height	Specify assessment, pre/post b'dilation exercise test etc	Wright PEF Meas.	Wright PEF Pred or best ever	Inhalation technique	Compliance	Days off school/work since last visit	**SYMPTOMS** (always check symptoms against the following list: cough, respiratory infection, bronchitis, sputum, exercise-induced asthma. Wheeziness worse at night and first thing in the morning?) HOME CHARTING RESULTS, EDUCATION, PLANS & THERAPY	APPT.

EDUCATION
Present level of understanding High / Med / Low Booklet given (Y/N) ❑

COMMENT and PLANS.......

Re-order this card (specify 'Gold Card R') from the NARTC, The Athenaeum, 10 Church Street, Warwick, CV34 4AB. Telephone (01926) 493313

Fig 5.3 Record card (front and back) designed and for sale by the National Asthma and Respiratory Training Centre, Warwick

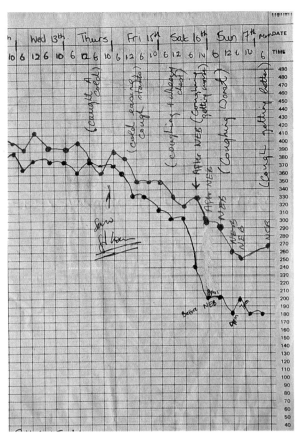

Figure 5.4 Peak flow chart demonstrating the danger of not taking early action

EXAMPLES OF PEAK FLOW CHARTS

Figure 5.4 This peak flow chart demonstrates the danger of not taking action early when readings start dropping. This asthmatic man with a history of previous severe attacks had been taught to monitor his peak flow readings and see his doctor if they changed. He went to his doctor on the Thursday with a history of an upper respiratory infection, increasing cough and a slight decline on his chart. In the absence of clinical signs, the doctor disagreed with the patient's request for oral steroids. Two days later his peak flow plummeted to 200 L/M and he was admitted to hospital where he required inpatient care for 29 days and oral steroids for nearly three months.

Figure 5.5 The use of predetermined 'action lines' in self-management plans is discussed in Chapter 6. This patient, a severe asthmatic child, had been given guidance to increase his inhaled steroids when the readings dropped below the first line, and to take oral prednisolone 15 mg bd when he dropped below the second. In the past he had been admitted to hospital with acute severe asthma on a number of occasions. The chart shows how the boy and his family were able to avert a potentially severe attack by following self-management advice.

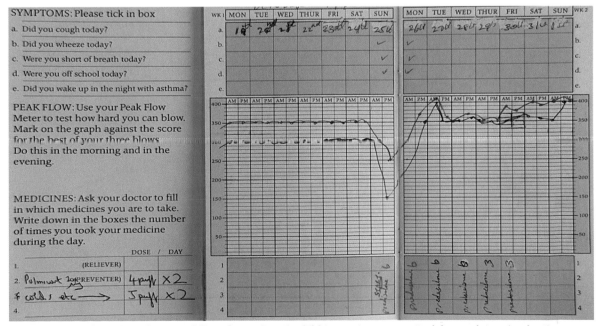

Figure 5.5 Peak flow chart showing ability of an asthmatic child to avert a severe attack by predetermined action

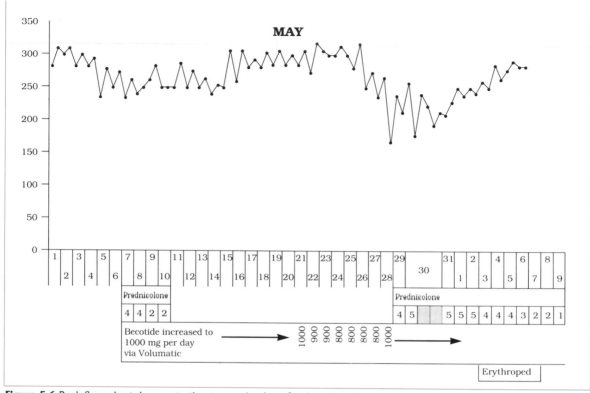

Figure 5.6 Peak flow chart demonstrating two episodes of asthma in a 7-year-old child

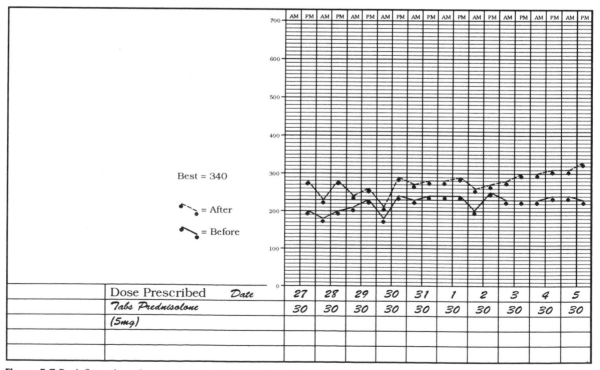

Figure 5.7 Peak flow chart demonstrating recovery phase following an acute attack

This family had instructions to contact the doctor if there were any problems. However, they felt in control of the situation and consulted only during the recovery phase of the attack.

Figure 5.6 This chart shows two episodes of uncontrolled asthma in a 7-year-old girl. The first was evident from the early morning dip from 290 to 230 L/M (26% variation) on 5 May. She had a short course of oral steroids and her beclomethasone was increased with a return to normal readings and reduction of symptoms by 17 May. Unfortunately, 12 days later she developed another episode, which was much more severe. This was resolved once again with oral steroids and, subsequently, antibiotics. This was in fact this child's seventh course of oral steroids in 11 months and she was referred to a paediatrician for advice on further management.

Figure 5.7 This patient, an 18-year-old female, presented on 27th of the month with acute asthma and the recovery phase of the attack is shown in the chart. There are three clear morning dips (>80%

variation from best), although the overall trend of the chart is increasing. It is interesting to note that after 13 days of oral steroids, there was still a variation of 17% before and after treatment.

Home peak flow charts can also be used when changing treatment or when trying to wean patients off therapy. A pattern of improvement, deterioration or constancy will usually be apparent. The opportunity for patient education by discussing therapy options, in conjunction with the peak flow chart, can be extremely helpful.

Figure 5.8 is a peak flow chart of an asthmatic adult with persistent symptoms. The readings appear fairly constant at around 300 L/M. Additional therapy was prescribed and his subsequent readings show a marked improvement of between 350 and 400 L/M.

The use of home peak flow recording in monitoring the progress of a patient during, and in the period following an acute severe attack, is dealt with in more detail in Chapter 6.

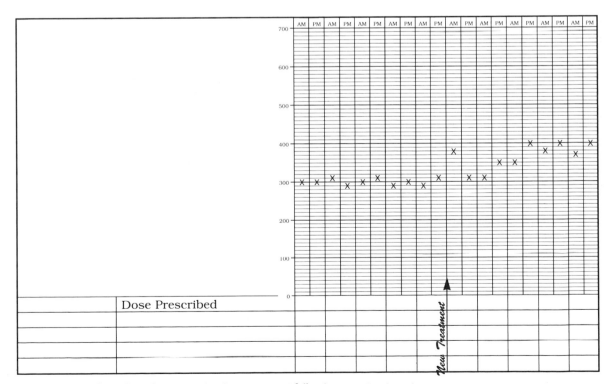

Figure 5.8 Peak flow chart demonstrating improvement following new treatment

Once uncontrolled asthma has been recognised, the next stage is to identify the reason(s). Common problems relate to the patient's understanding of the dosage and frequency of drugs, as well as the delivery device itself. The routine follow-up examination should be structured to detect the presence and nature of these problems. It is ultimately the responsibility of the prescribing clinician to ensure that the patient understands how to use the medication.

THE TREATMENT PATHWAY

The latest *British Asthma Guidelines* (The British Thoracic Society et al., 1997) have retained the stepwise approach (with slight modification) to drug management of asthma. The overall aim is to achieve best possible control of symptoms and lifestyle using the lowest drug dosage, with the least possible side effects. In general we use six groups of medication in managing asthma.

The following section is based on the published guidelines on the management of asthma (The British Thoracic Society et al., 1997). We refer the reader to the original guidelines for extra information. A summary of the British Guidelines is published every month in the MIMS magazine, available to all doctors in the UK (MIMS, 1998).

Initially, the British recommendation was to start at Step 1 (Anonymous, 1993) and progress up and down the steps depending upon the nature of the patient's symptoms and the peak flow readings at various stages of monitoring progress. The 1997 update suggested a 'start high' then step down approach. In other words, clinicians are advised to prescribe a high dose of inhaled or oral steroids and then to titrate the dose downwards once the patient improves, in terms of lung function and quality of life.

One of the greatest difficulties in following the stepwise plans, in the various guidelines, is the difficulty in deciding at what level to enter the patient. Dr Reggie Spelman, in the Irish College of General Practitioners' adaptation of the European Asthma Guidelines (Spelman, 1996), has made a useful suggestion to overcome this difficulty. Tables 5.1 and 5.2, reproduced from the Irish Guidelines, provide a framework for making this decision. He has combined features of history and examination with objective measures of lung function to provide a framework for deciding the level at which patients should be started (and subsequently varied at review assessments).

While the stepwise nature of the published guidelines is helpful, this process may result in over treatment through stepping up the treatment without subsequently modifying the doses according to the clinical response. An alternative approach is to think of the treatment pathway with more flexibility. A Canadian consensus conference (Ernst et al., 1996) devised the concept of the 'Asthma Continuum'. This advocates initial aggressive, high dose anti-inflammatory drug doses according to the frequency and chronicity of symptoms, the presence of airflow limitation and the medication required to maintain control of an individual patient. By titrating levels downward, control is then achieved with the lowest dose. The consensus for assessing asthma control was based on various parameters (listed in Table 5.3), with two outcomes: good control and acceptable control. This approach is a good one because poor control of asthma symptoms or lung function is not accepted; the clinician has two clear goals to aim for. This approach also has the advantage that the clinician does not have to guess which level to pitch initial treatment, but starts aggressively at a high level and works downwards to the lowest possible dose.

Parameters	Good control	Acceptable control
Daytime symptoms	None	<3 days/week
Night-time symptoms	Not woken	<1 night/week
Physical activity	Normal	Normal
Exacerbations	None	Mild, infrequent
Absenteeism	None	None
Need for prn beta-2 agonist	None*	<3 doses/week
FEV_1; FEV_1/FVC	Normal	90% personal best
PEF	Normal	90% personal best
PEF variability	<10% diurnal variation†	<15% diurnal variation
	5 days/week	5 days/week

FEV_1 Forced expiratory volume in 1 s; FVC Forced vital capacity obtained by spirometry; PEF Peak expiratory flow obtained with a portable peak flow meter. *May use one dose per day for prevention of exercise-induced symptoms; †Diurnal variation is calculated as the highest minus the lowest divided by the highest PEF multiplied by 100

Table 5.3 Criteria for asthma control

Source: reproduced with permission from Can Respir J Vol 3 No2 March/April 1996, page 91

Daytime symptoms cough/wheeze/dyspnoea	intermittent and < once a week	≥ once a week but < once a day	daily	continuous
Night-time symptoms cough/wheeze	< twice a month	> twice a month	> once a week *not every night*	*frequent or every night*
Limitation of activity due to exacerbation	never or occasional eg bad weather	sometimes	a lot of the time *but not continuous*	continuous
Inhaled short-acting B2 agonist use for symptom relief	< once a week intermittently	> once a week *but < once a day*	once daily	more than once a day
Highest peak flow reading over two weeks	≥ 80% of predicted	≥ 80% predicted	< 80% but > 60% predicted	≤ 60% predicted
Peak flow variability $\dfrac{highest - lowest}{highest} \times 100$	< 20%	20% - 30%	> 30%	> 30%
Asthma Severity (worst grade **any** feature is present)	Intermittent *(must be symptom free and have normal peak flow between exacerbations)*	mild persistent	moderate persistent	severe persistent
Treatment step	Step 1 oral steroids may be required for exacerbations	Step 2	Step 3 ? also start course of oral steroid	Step 4 Start with course of oral steroid

Table 5.1 First visit: grading asthma severity

Source: Spelman, 1996.

Daytime symptoms cough/wheeze/dyspnoea	< once a week	≥ once a week	continuous
Night-time symptoms cough/wheeze	<twice a month	> twice a month	> once a week
Limitation of activity Due to exacerbations	never	occasional	most of the time
Inhaled B2 agonist use for symptom relief	< once a week	> once a week but < once a day	every day
Highest peak flow reading over two weeks	≥ 80% of <u>best</u>	> 60% < 80%	< 60% of best
Peak flow variability $\dfrac{highest - lowest}{highest} \times 100$	≤20%	Best > 20% < 30%	> 30% of best
Control (worst level any feature is present)	good	poor	very poor/ no control
Treatment step	No change ? step down	If compliance and good inhaler technique confirmed, move up one step. ? also course of oral steroids	If compliance and good inhaler technique confirmed, move up one or two steps. Plus course of oral steroids

Table 5.2 Review visits: assessment of asthma control – based on past three months

Source: Spelman, 1996.

Indications for increasing medication include a history of increased need for inhaled rescue medication, symptoms of uncontrolled asthma as well as changes in peak flow readings (see earlier in this chapter). Symptoms that should prompt a move upwards include: night cough, wheeze or chest tightness, and exercise-induced symptoms. Increased diurnal variation in peak flow (by more than 15%) and early morning dipping on the peak flow chart are other objective criteria for increasing dosage or adding other medication.

It is advisable that inhaled steroids be prescribed to all patients from step two upwards. Other medication should be added to, rather than replace the use of inhaled topical steroids, because of the inflammatory nature of the disease and the proven benefit conferred by these drugs. This recommendation has been reinforced with regard to the long-acting beta-2 agonist bronchodilators because of possible extrapolation of data from studies on the short-acting beta-2 agonist bronchodilators. The issue arose a number of years ago in New Zealand with the association of increased mortality with the use of fenoterol. There was greater mortality in those patients using regular fenoterol, compared to those using the drug irregularly. One of the controversies was whether this was a phenomenon related specifically to fenoterol, or to the beta-2 bronchodilators in general. The Committee on Safety of Medicines (1992) stated that appropriate use of beta-2 agonist bronchodilators improves the quality of life of many asthmatic patients and that further clinical studies were required to resolve the controversy. The use of regular long-acting beta-2 agonist bronchodilators should be in addition to regular anti-inflammatory therapy, where this fails to control the asthma (British Thoracic Society, 1990; British Thoracic Society and others, 1993; Anonymous, 1993; Scheffer, 1995; Spelman, 1996; The British Thoracic Society et al., 1997).

Step 1. Short-acting beta-2 agonist bronchodilators

Short-acting beta-2 agonist bronchodilators (salbutamol 100-200 micrograms or terbutaline sulphate 250-500 microgrammes) should be used

> ### Drug management of asthma
>
> 1. Short-acting beta-2 agonist bronchodilators or relievers.
>
> 2. Anti-inflammatory drugs or preventers.
>
> 3. Long-acting beta-2 agonist bronchodilators.
>
> 4. Theophyllines.
>
> 5. Leucotriene receptor antagonist drugs (LTRAs).
>
> 6. Emergency drugs or acute savers which include oxygen, oral or parenteral steroids, and nebulised and parenteral bronchodilators.

as required, in response to symptom changes, rather than regularly. In mild asthmatics who have no sleep disturbance, infrequent symptoms, and whose peak flow readings remain constant, this may be all the treatment that is required. A patient's requirement to use these bronchodilators more than once a day indicates a need to step up treatment and seek medical advice.

In children under five years old, the medication should be administered via a large volume spacer with or without a mask (see Chapter 8).

Step 2. Inhaled anti-inflammatory agents

In view of the fact that asthma is a chronic inflammatory process, coupled with concerns regarding the use of regular short-acting beta-2 agonist bronchodilators, anti-inflammatory drugs are used as the mainstay of management (Committee on the Safety of Medicines, 1992). For adults, inhaled topical steroids are the drugs of choice at Step 2, and are indicated in those patients requiring inhaled beta-2 agonist bronchodilators more than once a day. In children there is an alternative choice of using cromoglycate at this step.

Three main inhaled topical steroid preparations are in use in the United Kingdom. These are:
1. Beclomethasone dipropionate (Becotide, Becloforte).
2. Budesonide (Pulmicort).
3. Fluticasone propionate (Flixotide).

Fluticasone propionate appears to combine high topical anti-inflammatory activity (Phillips, 1990), almost twice that of beclomethasone, with negligible oral systemic bioavailability (Harding, 1990). Consequently, this drug seems to have minimal potential for systemic side effects from the swallowed portion. Appropriate adult doses for beclomethasone dipropionate and budesonide in Step 2, range from 100-400ug twice daily and for fluticasone propionate the dose range is from 50-200mcg twice daily (half the corresponding beclomethasone dose). During times of uncontrolled asthma these doses may be stepped up for short periods of time. In children, half these doses are appropriate. There are a number of practical methods of using peak flow charts to determine when to adjust the dose of inhaled steroid (see Chapter 7).

Alternative anti-inflammatory drugs for adults are sodium cromoglycate (Intal) 520mg four times daily, and nedocromil sodium (Tilade) 4mg four times daily and the leucotriene receptor antagonist drugs (see below). While sodium cromoglycate has proved to be a milestone in treatment of asthmatic children, it is not often helpful in the management of adults.

Nedocromil sodium (Tilade) is positioned at Step 2 in the British Thoracic Society's guidelines, as an alternative to inhaled steroids, with the proviso that if control is not achieved, inhaled steroids should be started (British Thoracic Society and others, 1993; Anonymous, 1993; The British Thoracic Society et al., 1997). The main research findings of studies involving around 4,500 adult asthmatic patients have been elegantly summarised (Auty and Holgate, 1989) Nedocromil sodium was the first non-steroidal, broncho-specific anti-inflammatory drug designed for maintenance therapy for adult asthmatics. It has been shown to inhibit exercise-induced as well as allergen-induced immediate bronchoconstriction, and it was found to be more effective than placebo in the treatment of adult asthmatics. However, the authors concluded that the drug was *"unable to replace totally the use of inhaled steroids effectively in many patients"*. Some of the studies found that patients' asthma improved when nedocromil sodium was added to com-

bined inhaled steroids plus bronchodilator therapy. About 10% of adults react idiosyncratically with an unpleasant taste sensation, but there are no other reported significant side effects. Auty and Holgate (1989) suggested that this drug had potential as an adjunct to therapy with bronchodilators alone or in addition to inhaled steroids plus bronchodilators.

CFCs and HFAs (see Chapter 8)

It is common knowledge that the chlorofluorocarbons are being gradually phased out of use due to their adverse effects on the atmosphere. The pharmaceutical industry has excelled itself in working collaboratively to overcome this problem by identifying and producing an alternative propellant (Hydrofluoroalkane or HFA) for use in metered dose inhalers. 3M Pharmaceuticals has obtained a licence to market the first of these products in the UK, QVAR (beclomethasone dipropionate) and Airomir (salbutamol). Early studies indicate that the product QVAR (HFA beclomethasone) preparation is more efficient in its ability to penetrate the lungs and seems to be twice as effective clinically, when compared to the CFC product.

Literature and guidance on managing the transition to CFC free inhalers is available from some pharmaceutical companies and the National Asthma Campaign. While there is no immediate rush to switch patients to inhalers, the CFC to HFA transition has begun and licences to produce CFC inhalers will be granted once the alternatives are in place. All patients will need to be prescribed CFC free inhalers in the future. We suggest that newly diagnosed people with asthma could be prescribed a CFC free inhaler, patients who attend the surgery or clinic could be switched if they need a repeat prescription and when there is no longer an alternative, the rest of the patients could be recalled.

Step 3. Inhaled topical steroids plus adjuvant therapy

If asthma is not controlled at Step 2 (and compliance or poor inhaler technique are not responsible), the patient should try high dose inhaled steroids. Beclomethasone dipropionate or budesonide in doses of 800-2000mcg daily should be administered via a large spacer device. The spacer reduces systemic absorption and local side effects, such as oral thrush and hoarseness. The Volumatic is appropriate for beclomethasone and fluticasone, while the Nebuhaler is used for budesonide. Fluticasone propionate can be used at doses of 400-1,000mcg daily in this step. Studies have shown that fluticasone, delivered through a dry powdered device, induces no more local side effects than beclomethasone delivered either directly through an aerosol or a large volume spacer.

Clinicians should be aware that the British Guidelines on chronic asthma care for children over five years old were included in the same section as for adults guidelines (Chart 1, page S11, The British Thoracic Society et al., 1997). It is clearly inadvisable to prescribe inhaled steroid doses, at Steps 3 and 4, up to 2,000mcg in a six year old. Thus, the doses recommended were too high for this age group. Children under 15 years old should not be prescribed the high doses recommended in Chart 1 of the 1995 guidelines (The British Thoracic Society et al., 1997) unless they have been advised to do so by a respiratory paediatrician (personal communication Dr Warren Lenney, paediatrician).

For those patients not controlled on these doses there are three therapy options (also see box):
1. The addition of a long-acting beta-2 agonist bronchodilator, a theophylline preparation or a leucotriene receptor antagonist.
2. Increase to Step 4 by doubling the dose of inhaled topical steroids.
3. If the additional medication fails to control the patients' asthma, the dose of inhaled topical steroids can be increased as well as adding one of the preparations mentioned above.

For those who cannot tolerate increased doses of inhaled topical steroids for various reasons (mainly side effects such as hoarseness), the first of these should be pursued.

Guidelines are not absolute, and there are situations where strict adherence may not resolve the patients' symptoms or improve lung function. It is important to incorporate the patient's clinical response when making any changes to the man-

---

1. BDP/BUD 200-800 OR FP 50-200 plus LABag, Theophylline or a leucotriene receptor antagonist drug.
2. Double ITS/(BDP/BUD) 800-2000 OR FP to 400-1000.
3. Add (II) plus increase ITS (ie go to Step 4).

Key
BDP Beclomethasone dipropionate
BUD Budesonide
LABag Long-acting beta agonist bronchodilators
FP Fluticasone propionate
LTRA Leucotriene receptor antagonist

---

agement plan. A clinical review should probably occur a suitable time after adjusting or adding medication. The 'suitable time' would depend on the stability or severity of the patient's asthma. For example, a person with wide variations in PEF, or who is waking at night due to asthma, may need a short course of oral steroids and daily review until resolved. Alternatively, someone at Step 2, who has been experiencing slight increases in symptoms may be reassessed a month after the addition of a long-acting beta-2 agonist bronchodilator.

Since the publication of the British Guidelines two of the leucotriene receptor antagonists and synthesis inhibitor (LTRAs) drugs have been licensed for prescription in the UK. These are montelukast (Singulair) and zafirlukast (Accolate). The cysteinyl-leukotrienes (LTC4, LTD4 and LTE4) are produced by many of the inflammatory cells involved in asthma, and are released by a variety of asthma triggers. Studies have shown that the leukotrienes contribute to the resting tone of asthmatic airways and play a key role in bronchospasm, induced by various triggers of asthma such as allergen, exercise, and aspirin.

The leukotrienes modify airways responsiveness in a number of ways:

1. They produce bronchoconstriction.
2. They increase airway mucus secretion and microvascular permeability, leading to mucosal oedema.
3. They stimulate release or potentiate the effects of other inflammatory mediators.

Leucotriene receptor antagonist drugs (information prepared by the NARTC, Warwick)

- different class of drug
- blocks or prevents inflammatory leucotriene mediators
- inhibits early and late response
- additional therapy to inhaled anti-inflammatory drugs
- effective in people who are allergic to aspirin

Currently, there are very few published studies on the LTRA drugs. Montelukast (Singulair) was the first to be licensed for prescription in the United Kingdom. It is prescribed as chewable 5mg and 10mg tablets. The drug is indicated for addition to inhaled steroid therapy of asthma in adults (15 years and older) at 10mg daily, and in children aged 6 to 14 years at 5mg daily (Reiss and et al., 1998; Reiss et al., 1997). LTRAs are at least partially independent of inhaled steroids, and in the case of aspirin sensitive patients, the level of benefit is even independent of whether patients are taking oral steroids.

Zafirlukast was licensed in 1998 in the UK for treatment of asthma in people over the age of 12 years. It is prescribed in tablet form, 20mg bd for adult asthma. In a multicentre, randomised placebo-controlled parallel group study in 762 people with mild to moderate asthma, the drug was significantly better than placebo in improving quality of life and lung function (Fish et al., 1997). Another, smaller study showed that the drug is better than placebo in mild to moderate asthma when added to 'as needed' beta-2 agonist bronchodilator (Suissa et al., 1997). Initial abstract data on the comparative efficacy of zafirlukast and beclomethasone dipropionate indicate, a slight advantage in favour of BDP (Laitinen et al., 1997). Since releasing the drug in the USA, where it has been used quite extensively, a number of cases of Churg-Strauss Syndrome (also known as allergic angiitis and granulomatosis) have been reported, associated with a reduction in oral steroid dosage coincident with prescription of zafirlukast. It is not known whether the syndrome is caused by zafirlukast or whether it is revealed as a consequence of reduction in steroid doses. Clinicians are advised to monitor closely those patients reducing their oral steroid dosage. Furthermore, drug interactions occur with warfarin, terfenadine and erythromycin. Reports of elevated liver enzymes in patients receiving high dosages of zafirlukast (80mg twice daily) preclude the use of dosages exceeding 40mg twice daily.

In summary, zafirlukast is a potentially useful addition to current anti-asthma therapies in patients with mild to moderate asthma. Because it is administered orally, it may be particularly beneficial in those patients with a poor inhaler technique and do not respond to further instruction.

It seems that these drugs may have an important role in the future management of asthma, particularly because of the apparent inability of inhaled steroids to block fully mediator production - hence the demonstration of the LTRA 'add-on' effect. However, given the available data at the time of writing, it is advisable that these drugs should be used as add-on therapy to inhaled steroids preferably at level 3 or level 2 in cases where increased doses of inhaled steroids are not possible. In our view, there is insufficient evidence at present to justify prescribing these drugs instead of inhaled steroids at level 2.[†]

Salmeterol and efformoterol are effective for at least 12 hours and are therefore convenient for patients to use at the same time as the inhaled topical steroids. It is also important to note that the regular use of the short-acting beta-2 agonist bronchodilators (salbutamol or terbutaline) should be discontinued when initiating salmeterol or eformoterol, otherwise the patient will lose the advantage of recognising the need for having rescue medication when trouble arises.

The other options in this step are the xanthines, ipatropium bromide, long-acting oral bronchodilator, bambuterol (active for 24 hours) and high dose bronchodilators via a nebuliser or large spacer device. Oral bronchodilators (short-acting or long-acting beta-2 agonists) are sometimes of help especially for those patients who have night symptoms. However, in our experi-

[†]We thank Dr David Price, Norwich, for his assistance in preparing this section on LTRA drugs

ence many patients complain of side effects such as palpitations and cramps and therefore these oral drugs should only be used if the inhaled route is not acceptable.

Methylxanthines are more popular in other countries than in the UK. These drugs are recommended as additional therapy at Step 4. However, methylxanthines are used with patients who react adversely to inhaled steroids (The British Thoracic Society et al., 1997). Gastrointestinal side effects are common and irritability is a problem, especially in younger patients. Complications related to the use of these drugs include convulsions, cardiac arrythmias and even death. The main problems relate to interactions with other drugs (erythromycin, cimetidine) and accidental overdoses resulting from bolus injections in patients on oral methylxanthine preparation. Serum level monitoring is recommended for patients prescribed these drugs on a regular basis.

Ipatropium bromide, an anticholinergic preparation, has long been used as an adjunct to other anti-asthma therapy in the older asthmatic patient. It is useful in those patients who have a degree of chronic obstructive airways disease in addition to their asthma. Many patients find the side effects of this drug (dryness of the mouth, tachycardia, irritability and tremors) intolerable. An alternative anticholinergic drug, oxitropium bromide, is administered twice daily and is claimed to be more effective than ipatropium in the maintenance of chronic asthma in adults.

Step 4. High dose inhaled steroids
At this step, patients are prescribed doses of inhaled beclomethasone or budesonide inhaled steroids ranging from 400 to 1,000mcg twice daily, or fluticasone between 200 and 500mcg twice daily. At this step any of the additional preparations may be added.

Step 5. Long-term maintenance therapy with oral steroids
We believe that those few patients who require long-term oral steroids should be under the supervision of an asthma specialist.

CONCLUSION
Asthma is so variable within and between patients that clinicians need to adopt a flexible approach to implementing guidelines and protocols. Assessment of the patient's clinical response to therapy is ultimately the best determinant of effective therapy.

6

UNCONTROLLED AND ACUTE SEVERE ASTHMA

INTRODUCTION

Episodes of acute asthma may be viewed as a failure of management on the part of health professionals. Patients themselves bear some responsibility for recognising and acting upon the early warning signs of an impending attack, provided they have been informed previously.

Research papers on deaths from asthma, provide much of the evidence relating to the management of acute asthma; therefore this chapter discusses some of these studies. By addressing the conclusions and recommendations from these studies, it is possible to modify the management of acute asthma in the community.

Despite the puzzling variation in rates for asthma world wide, the circumstances surrounding deaths from acute asthma are very similar. They include a failure by doctors, people with asthma and their relatives, to recognise the severity of acute asthma attacks as well as a failure to treat these attacks appropriately (Stableforth, 1993; Priel, 1993; Fletcher et al., 1990; Levy, 1988; Eason and Markowe, 1987; Asthma mortality task force (1986), 1987; British Thoracic Association, 1982). Furthermore, many of the asthma deaths reported are still believed to have been preventable; a recent confidential Scottish report revealed that 30% of asthma related deaths were associated with poor management.

In the last decade, there was concern about the relationship between regular use of short-acting beta-2 agonist bronchodilator drugs (Rea et al., 1986; Beasley et al., 1994) and deaths from asthma probably linked to the use of fenoterol. Although the evidence indicates strongly that the beta-2 agonist related deaths were associated with a specific drug effect due to fenoterol, there does remain some controversy whether this was in fact a class effect related to short-acting beta-2 agonist drugs in general (Garrett et al., 1996; Fuller, 1996). Sears concluded (Sears, 1995) on the basis of the evidence from these and other studies, that patients were more likely to develop deterioration in asthma control, with increased morbidity and mortality, if prescribed regular versus intermittent (rescue) use of short-acting beta-2 agonists. As a result, UK and International asthma guidelines (British Thoracic Society and others, 1993; Anonymous, 1993; Scheffer, 1995; The British Thoracic Society et al., 1997) have all stressed that short-acting beta-2 agonist bronchodilators (such as salbutamol and terbutaline) should only be used as intermittent, rescue therapy. Any patient requiring one or more doses of these drugs per day should be prescribed an anti-inflammatory drug (such as an inhaled topical steroid, sodium cromoglycate, or nedocromil sodium).

What can be done?

The fact that many deaths from asthma are still thought to be avoidable should lead to a modification of approach to the management of acute asthma. While at-risk registers may be helpful in identifying those in danger of asthma death, there is no guarantee that doctors treating patients will be aware of their 'at-risk' status. Furthermore, with few exceptions, most studies have failed to identify reliable risk factors for asthma death. McFadden (McFadden Jr and Warren, 1997), in a helpful recent review, stated that all exacerbations of asthma that last longer than a few days (particularly in those who had had a severe episode of asthma in the past) should be regarded as potentially fatal. This book goes a step further than this and advises that all episodes of uncontrolled asthma should be taken very seriously indeed and treated as emergencies in the pre-hospital setting. A rational, methodical approach to managing acute asthma would help to ensure the best possible outcome for each patient.

1. Diagnosis of acute asthma

Strictly speaking, uncontrolled episodes of asthma are asthma attacks. For the purpose of clarity, in this chapter we refer to these episodes of poor control as 'asthma attacks'; the assessed severity of these attacks determines the level of management. The principles of diagnosis of asthma attacks are similar to those used when initially diagnosing asthma. Worrying symptoms, a requirement for rescue medication and significant variability of lung function in someone previously diagnosed with asthma are signs of inadequate control.

An integrated approach to early recognition, diagnosis and management of asthma attacks is required. This involves co-operation between all those involved in the management of asthma. Patients need to be taught how to recognise when to initiate rescue medication and to call for help. Surgery reception staff need to be aware of the procedures for 'fast tracking' patients with acute asthma and the doctor or nurse has to make a rapid assessment of the severity of the episode in order to initiate appropriate management rapidly.

Diagnosis and initial management by the patient

Self-management plans (SMPs) are now accepted as part of the usual management package for asthma. There is evidence of their effectiveness and they are recommended in the majority of published guidelines on asthma management (see SMPs in Chapter 7). They may be simple or quite elaborate. A self-management plan enables patients to monitor their asthma control, through subjective or objective measures, coupled with instructions on when and how to adjust medication and to call for help.

Figure 6.1 shows a personally tailored self-management plan devised by a nurse for a patient. The nurse has drawn 'action lines' on the chart (80% – yellow and 60% – orange of best PEF) in order to assist the patient in deciding when to increase the dose of inhaled steroid, add oral steroid or to call for help.

The best ever peak expiratory flow is used as the patient's 'normal'; this is determined from the average best readings taken when the patient is well or on a short course of oral steroids. Two 'action lines' are then drawn across the peak flow chart, one at the 80% level and one at the 60% level, simply calculated by multiplying the best PEF by 0.8 and 0.6 respectively (Figure 6.1). The patient is advised to measure the peak flow twice a day (best of three) and aim to keep the level above the 80% line. Advice is tailored to the PEF readings, and as these drop towards the action lines, patients will initiate certain pre-arranged self-treatment options (written down) by the doctor or nurse. For example, if the read-

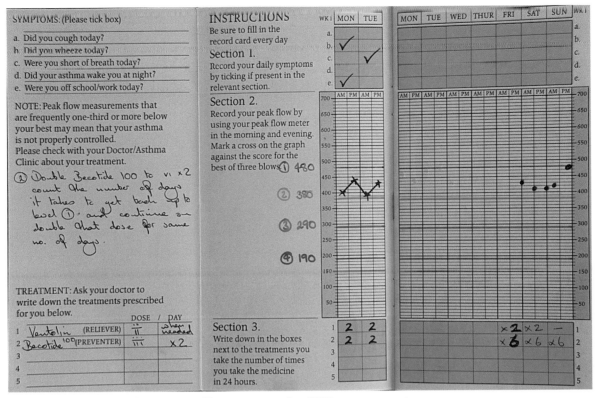

Figure 6.1 An example of an asthma self-management plan (SMP)

ings approach or drop below the top action line, the patient would increase their use of reliever as well as double their inhaled steroid treatment. If the readings approach or drop below the lower line the patient would also initiate a short course of oral steroids. Once the PEF readings have returned to normal (usual best) then the patient should 'step down' the therapy to the lowest possible dose required for adequate control.

Another aspect of the SMP includes patients' recognising that an increase in asthma symptoms or a requirement for using a short-acting beta-2 agonist bronchodilator, constitute a need for additional treatment. Detailed instruction should also be provided on increasing medication if asthma symptoms become troublesome and then reducing once control has been achieved.

Providing patients with the ability to monitor their asthma and to adjust medication when necessary does carry significant responsibility. Safeguards need to be built into the system in order to protect patients. Particular danger signs need to be made

explicit and patients should be in no doubt about when and how to seek medical assistance.

They need to be clear which drug is for emergency (rescue) use. They should be taught to increase their usual beta-2 agonist bronchodilator at the first sign of deterioration of their asthma (symptoms or peak flow rates). They should also know that it is safe to use these short-acting bronchodilators in large doses, which may be delivered via a large volume spacer device or simply by means of a paper coffee cup with a hole cut in the base (Henry et al., 1983). Home nebulisers driven by air, are not advisable for patient use in view of the theoretical risk of precipitating life threatening hypoxia due to ventilation perfusion inequality (see later in this chapter). Uncertainty regarding the dose to be given in these circumstances can be overcome by advising patients to use four puffs of their short-acting bronchodilator (used one at a time) via a large volume spacer, every ten minutes, until relief is obtained or medical help arrives (Cates, 1998).

Patients should be aware of the following:

1. Short-acting beta-2 agonist bronchodilators should give quick relief from asthma and that this relief should last for four hours. If not, help should be sought.

2. Once help has been sought, short-acting beta-2 agonist bronchodilators are required and safe to use in episodes of severe asthma, sometimes in very high doses while awaiting arrival of medical or paramedic help.

3. A drop in PEF to below 30% of usual best level, an inability to speak in sentences, a blue discoloration of the lips, tongue or skin constitutes a medical emergency and assistance should be sought immediately.

The severity of asthma varies from one patient to another, therefore SMPs need to be individually tailored. Practices may aim for better control of their patients' asthma by calculating different 'action levels'. For example an 85% and a 65% level.

Once the patient is familiar with the SMP, there may be no need to contact the doctor, provided there are clear instructions for recognising worsening asthma. It is not necessary to wean the patient off a short course of oral prednisolone. It is safe to stop this suddenly provided the course duration is under two weeks.

Diagnosis by the practice staff

The receptionist and practice nurse may recognise those patients requesting extra bronchodilator prescriptions; these should be invited to see the doctor or nurse urgently. The whole practice team, including the health visitor, district nurse and the reception staff, should be aware of the severe danger signs of impending acute asthma; protocols should be in place in order to ensure urgent treatment.

Diagnosis of acute asthma by the doctor or nurse

Uncontrolled asthma should be considered in any previously diagnosed asthma patient who consults with respiratory symptoms such as cough, wheeze or shortness of breath. A common mistake, when consulted, is to misdiagnose the symptoms of an asthma exacerbation as infection. Although acute asthma exacerbations may begin insidiously, they can progress very rapidly to a life threatening situation. The history and examination may lead to a diagnosis of uncontrolled asthma. Home peak flow recordings provide additional information; some patients may not volunteer this. The episode may have been precipitated by trigger factors known to the patient but it is necessary to take a detailed history to determine whether other factors, such as exposure to household or occupational triggers, may have been responsible. Physical examination of the respiratory system, together with objective measures of lung function, will help to confirm the diagnosis.

An example of clear written instructions detailing how patients should implement their SMP:

"If the peak flow rate drops below the top line then double the dose of your inhaled steroid (eg beclomethasone, budesonide or fluticasone). Continue taking this dose until the peak flow reaches the previous 'normal' level. Count the number of days it took to get back to this level and continue taking the increased dose for the same number of days. If the peak flow stays at your normal level for a few days, then reduce your inhaled steroid to the usual dose.

If the peak flow level drops below the lower line, start taking (Xmg) oral steroids, ie prednisolone (12mg Kg/day, maximum 40mg for children, and maximum 60mg for adults) and contact the doctor or practice nurse. Continue at that dose until the previous 'normal' level is attained. Then count the number of days it took and continue on half the dose of oral steroids for the same number of days."

2. The assessment of the severity of the attack – treatment, monitoring and decision regarding admission[†]

Having diagnosed acute asthma a clinician is faced with decisions related to the immediate management of the attack and whether the patient requires referral to hospital for admission. The severity of the attack needs to be established very early in order to decide to refer the patient and to initiate a request for ambulance paramedic assistance. It is essential to adopt a management approach that ensures a constant rapidly repeated cycle of assessment, treatment and recognition of markers of severity. The British Guidelines on asthma management have defined clear criteria for assessing the severity, as well as treating and admitting patients with acute asthma attacks.

The following two tables (see Tables 6.1 and 6.2) have been summarised and adapted from the British Guidelines (The British Thoracic Society et al., 1997) and are of assistance in the rapid assessment of the severity of an attack.

	Children under 5 years	Children 5 to 15 years
Breathing	Too breathless to talk or feed Use of accessory muscles ie alae nasi, scaleni, sternocleidomastoid and intercostal muscles	
Respiratory rate	> 50 per minute	> 40 per minute
Pulse rate	> 140 per minute	> 120 per minute
Pulse oximetry; oxygen saturation (SaO2)	< 92%	< 92%
Peak Expiratory Flow (PEF)		< 50% predicted or Best
Life threatening features	Cyanosis, silent chest or poor respiratory effort	PEF < 33% predicted or best
	Fatigue or exhaustion	Cyanosis, silent chest or poor respiratory effort
	Agitation or reduced level of consciousness	Fatigue or exhaustion
		Agitation or reduced level of consciousness

Table 6.1 Acute severe asthma in children

Source: The British Thoracic Society et al., 1997.

	Uncontrolled asthma	Acute severe	Life threatening
Breathing	Speech normal	Can't complete sentences	Silent chest Cyanosis Exhaustion
Respiratory rate (per minute)	< 25	>25	Slow
Pulse rate	< 110	> 110	Bradycardia
Refer for blood gas analysis	If SaO2 is < 92%		
Peak Expiratory Flow (PEF) (% predicted or best)	> 50%	< 50%	< 33%

Table 6.2 Acute asthma in adults in primary care

Source: The British Thoracic Society et al., 1997.

[†]The following paragraphs and two tables were first published in the Members' Reference Book 1998/99, Levy M (1998), and have been reproduced with permission of the publisher, Campden Publishing Ltd, London.

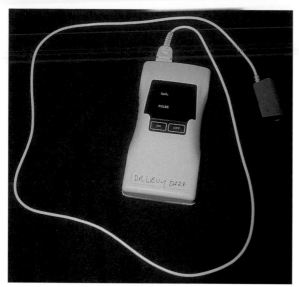

Figure 6.2 Pulse oximeter - a non invasive method of assessment

Pulse and respiratory rates, coupled with observations regarding patients' use of accessory muscles of respiration, offer a means of assessing the nature of an attack. Decreased or variable measurements of PEF or FEV₁ offer further objective information regarding the severity of an asthma attack. Another measurement, pulse oximetry, is extremely useful before, during and after treatment of an acute attack. Pulse oximetry is not yet used widely in primary care, but it does have a role in determining whether to admit a patient, initially treated in primary care, to hospital. In addition, this provides very valuable information in those unable or too ill to perform a PEF manoeuvre. Pulse oximeters offer a non-invasive, useful and affordable measurement of the efficacy of respiration (see Figure 6.2).

Geelhoed and colleagues (Geelhoed et al., 1994) have demonstrated that the pre-treatment oxygen saturation (SaO2) is useful in establishing the severity of a childhood asthma attack – thus providing predictive information on the probable effectiveness of treatment and the need for specialist referral. Children with pre-treatment levels below 91% are associated with high risk, requiring intravenous treatment and hospital admission. This predictive quality of SaO2 is independent of current or past clinical factors and therefore provides the clinician with a useful near patient test, informing management decisions in the pre-hospital setting.

Monitoring during the management of an asthma attack should be done regularly (probably every five minutes) and recorded. An example of a flow sheet for this purpose is illustrated in Table 6.3; this may be helpful in determining whether to admit a patient. The flow sheet can also serve as an objective record for hospital staff and would help their decision on whether to treat the patient in hospital and if so, for how long. One of the most frustrating situations for primary care health workers occurs when acute asthma patients are prematurely sent home from hospital. This suggested approach might help to inform junior hospital doctors and assist them in the management of these at-risk patients.

Treatment of the attack

Treatment for acute asthma includes short-acting beta-2 agonist bronchodilators, oxygen and steroids. The British Guidelines (The British Thoracic Society et al., 1997) make different recommendations for the delivery of bronchodilators in the management of acute severe asthma in primary and secondary care. For hospital treatment, oxygen-driven nebulised bronchodilators are recommended, while general practitioners are advised to use either a nebuliser or a spacer device to administer bronchodilators. While it is clear that an oxygen-driven nebulised bronchodilator is the gold standard, there is some evidence to suggest that these drugs are as effective when delivered via spacers.

There are three issues for debate:
• should nebulisers be driven by air or oxygen?
• are spacers as effective as air-driven nebulisers?
• are spacers as effective as oxygen-driven nebulisers?

Cates published a systematic review comparing spacers and nebulisers for treating acute asthma (Cates, 1998). The review summarised and discussed 13 papers (of the 113 published to date on this subject) which were considered relevant for inclusion. His main conclusions were:

1. There was no significant difference in hospital admission rates when the two delivery methods were compared.

Name: .... DOB: ..../................/................

Date: .... / .... /................ Time first seen: .... H ....

History:..
....

Time	Pulse rate	Respiratory rate	Using accessory	Pulse oximetry muscles	Cyanosis	Exhaustion	Oxygen flow rate	Treatment
...... H.........			SCM y/n Scaleni y/n Alae nasi y/n Intercostals y/n				___L/M	Salbutamol/ Terbutaline Dose: _____ Delivery: Nebuliser/Spacer Oral Steroid:_____ Inhaled Steroid: _____
...... H.........			SCM y/n Scaleni y/n Alae nasi y/n Intercostals y/n				___L/M	Salbutamol/ Terbutaline Dose: _____ Delivery: Nebuliser/Spacer Oral Steroid:_____ Inhaled Steroid: _____
...... H.........			SCM y/n Scaleni y/n Alae nasi y/n Intercostals y/n				___L/M	Salbutamol/ Terbutaline Dose: _____ Delivery: Nebuliser/Spacer Oral Steroid:_____ Inhaled Steroid: _____

Table 6.3 Monitoring chart for acute asthma attacks treated in the pre-hospital setting

SCM = Sternocleidomastoid muscles

2. Children spent less time in Accident and Emergency departments if spacers were used.
3. pMDIs with spacers, produced outcomes that were at least equivalent to nebuliser delivery of beta-2 agonist bronchodilator in acute asthma.

Cates raised several issues restricting the generalisability of those studies reviewed:

1. For adults, seen and assessed for acute exacerbations of asthma, this review found no significant differences between the two delivery methods. Consequently, Cates suggested that the choice of delivery method could reflect patient preference, practice situations and formal economic evaluation.
2. In children, no outcomes were significantly worse with the spacers. The available evidence suggested that, in most cases, spacers could be substituted for nebulisers to deliver beta-2 agonist bronchodilator to acute asthma patients in emergency departments.

3. The experimental method adopted in many of the studies gave repeated treatments at short intervals (eg one respule via a nebuliser or four actuations of a metered-dose inhaler via a holding chamber every 15 minutes). The number of treatments required was adjusted to the individual patient's response, overcoming the uncertainty of dosage delivery from different devices. This method of dosing is therefore recommended for practice until further evidence becomes available.
4. The studies excluded patients with life threatening asthma; therefore, the results of this meta-analysis should not be extrapolated to this patient population.

While this review was thorough, and is currently accepted as the best evidence on the subject of delivery of bronchodilators to patients suffering from acute asthma, we urge some caution in the applicability of these data to the primary care setting. The studies reviewed by Cates:

1. Excluded severe asthma attacks and were unclear regarding the selection of patients for study.

2. 13 were hospital-based (all but one) and therefore included patients who may or may not have been treated in primary care, or by ambulance paramedic staff en route to the hospital; this could clearly have affected the outcome.

3. In the case of three of the seven paediatric studies, oxygen-driven nebulisers were used to deliver bronchodilators.

4. Did not provide much data on the outcome for patients after being treated and discharged from the hospitals.

All of these factors are relevant to the management choices in primary care.

Furthermore, two studies investigating the effect of air-driven nebulised bronchodilators (Douglas et al., 1985) and comparing air-driven with oxygen-driven nebulisers (Gleeson et al., 1988) highlighted important safety issues. Four out of 32 adults in one study (Douglas et al., 1985) and 10 out of 27 children in the other (Gleeson et al., 1988) deteriorated significantly soon after initiating the nebulisers. While the group mean SaO2 in this study did not fall significantly, some children deteriorated markedly. It is impossible to predict who is going to deteriorate and it would therefore seem safer to use oxygen as a driving gas for nebulisers and as routinely available therapy in the case of acute attacks. In a primary care setting, in the event of a delay in obtaining assistance from the ambulance paramedic service, a patient who deteriorates with therapy could pose a very tricky problem for the health professional concerned.

In the current absence of relevant primary care data on the type of patients treated for acute asthma in this setting, there are a limited number of delivery options for bronchodilators. Of the choices available, the best option would be to use oxygen-driven nebulised bronchodilators for acute asthma. This would necessitate the availability of oxygen cylinders fitted with a high flow regulator (delivering up to 15 litres per minute, see Figure 6.3). Oxygen may be purchased by general practitioners in the UK at an annual cost of about £150. With the establishment of co-operatives as the predominant out-of-hours model of care in general practice, this suggestion is more realistic than it would have been in the past. The next best option would seem to be the use of a spacer device together with a pMDI to deliver a short-acting beta-2 agonist bronchodilator. Whichever method is used, short bursts of therapy should be frequent, titrated against the patients' clinical response (see Table 6.4).

Oral steroids

There is no advantage to be gained by administering cortisone by injection unless the patient is unable to swallow medication. This was demonstrated in a prospective study comparing oral with intravenous prednisolone in 77 patients with acute severe asthma (Ratto et al., 1988). Prescribe sufficient prednisolone tablets (soluble for children) to cover the time interval to the review appointment if not admitting the patient. Recommended dosage is 12mg/Kg/day for children (maximum 40mg/day), and 30-60mg/day for adults. Adults may take the dose once daily after meals; divided doses would be more appropriate for children.

Deciding whether to admit patients with acute asthma

Any patient with life threatening features of acute asthma should be admitted to hospital (see Tables 6.1 and 6.2). By monitoring patients as described above, it should become clear, fairly quickly, if a patient is deteriorating or failing to improve. These patients need to be admitted to hospital.

Drug	Dose
Salbutamol pMDI*	20-50 puffs (25 g)
Nebuliser	2.5-10 mg
Terbutaline Inhaler*	10-20 puffs (2.55 mg)
Nebuliser	2-10 mg

* According to Cates, four puffs (one at a time) were administered via a large volume spacer every 15 minutes. The British Guidelines however, suggest one puff every 15 seconds. Until further evidence is available, we recommend that readers use their clinical judgement and administer one puff of beta-2 agonist bronchodilator via a large volume spacer every 15 seconds until the patient is relieved or help arrives.

Table 6.4 Emergency dose of short-acting beta-2 agonists in asthma

Protocols

Protocols provide guidance for all members of the primary health care team as well as the patients themselves. These can be developed by individual practices; please see Appendix 1 for an outline protocol which can be modified to suit individual needs. The protocols should be available to locums if the usual doctor is away, to new partners, nurses and registrars when they join the practice. Locate the protocol in the treatment room, with copies in the doctors' bags so that it is accessible when having to deal with an emergency situation. The flow charts available within the British Guidelines are useful for this purpose.

3. After the attack – therapy and follow-up

Of patients who die from asthma, a high proportion suffer a fatal relapse during the three month period following an attack. Therefore, recovering patients *must* be monitored to ensure their symptoms and lung function have stabilised, and that the attack has resolved fully. Another major reason for follow-up assessment is to advise the patient how and when to reduce medication to pre-attack levels, if appropriate.

There are two possible scenarios: patients who have been treated in hospital for their asthma, and patients treated entirely in the community. A systematic approach would ensure adequate follow-up for those people treated in hospital; either by the hospital or the primary care team. Some hospital departments arrange follow-up appointments while others do not. In either event, we suggest that the practices arrange follow-up appointments for all patients suffering acute attacks, irrespective of where they were treated.

Those people, treated by the primary care team who have improved satisfactorily following treatment, should be sent home with a peak flow meter and advice to chart the measurements every 2 to 4 hours, at least for the first 48 hours. Written guidelines, indicating clearly when the patient should contact the doctor, are important because a distressed patient or parent may not be able to remember verbal advice.

There is no need to tail the dose of prednisolone gradually, provided that the duration of this therapy is under two weeks.

We believe that patients who suffer an acute severe attack of asthma should be prescribed an inhaled topical steroid (if not already on this). However, it is debatable whether this should be added at the time of the prescription of the short course of oral steroids, or at the review appointment the next day. The aim of early introduction of inhaled topical steroids is to try and reduce the length of time required for oral prednisolone.

Advise the patient to make an appointment for the next day, to be seen by either the doctor or asthma nurse, and to contact the doctor urgently if there is any deterioration (either clinical or from the peak flow readings).

Review the patient the next day and then every few days until the symptoms have cleared and the peak flow rates are satisfactory. The use of peak flow charts in monitoring the progress of acute attacks enable doctors and nurses to decide objectively when the oral steroids can be stopped or reduced. In this way, the problems of either using too much steroid or stopping too soon are avoided. The patient should also be advised to continue to use the rescue bronchodilator every four hours as needed during the recovery phase

---

Follow-up after an asthma attack

1. Identify those patients who have been treated for asthma attacks (in a practice or hospital).
2. Ensure they are seen (by the doctor or asthma nurse) within a day or two of the attack.
3. Peak flow meters for those older than five years.
4. Prescribe sufficient prednisolone (soluble for children) to continue; and issue steroid cards.
5. Provide self-management plans.
6. Continue follow-up until the attack has resolved (ie symptoms, use of rescue beta-2 agonist bronchodilators and PEF variability).
7. Add a topical inhaled steroid if not already prescribed.

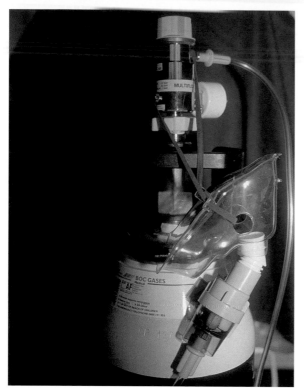

Figure 6.3 High flow oxygen regulator - providing the ability to deliver oxygen and drive a nebuliser up to flow rates between one and 15 L/M

of the attack. The difficult decision on when to reduce the oral steroids is made easier by developing a logical approach to the problem. Beasley suggested halving the daily dose of oral steroids once the patient's daily peak flow recording reaches the normal level. This is continued for the same number of days that it took to recover (Beasley et al., 1989).

Plans for the long-term follow-up could then be based upon the severity of the asthma. One of the problems facing doctors in managing acute asthma, is the intra-patient and inter-patient variability of these attacks. There are many anecdotal tales of the different regimes used for short courses of oral steroids. How can one know exactly when an acute episode is going to resolve? Without objective measurements, the timing of resolution of an attack is guesswork. Despite the availability of cheap peak flow meters, they have not been used to their full potential. Measurement of patients' peak flow rates, even during hospital admission for acute asthma, has been shown to vary markedly. Several studies of deaths from asthma have concluded that use of peak flow meters fell far short of acceptable levels. Now that they are available on prescription in the UK there shouldn't be a reason not to use them.

Once the patient's peak flow rate has reached acceptable levels (within 70% to 85% of the best or normal levels), further arrangements for the doctor or nurse to see the patient for review is advisable. Bucknall showed that many patients in the group of acute asthmatics studied were still suffering from incapacitating symptoms 13 days after hospital discharge (Bucknall et al., 1988b). In a randomised, double blind study, Levy compared high dose inhaled with oral steroids for acute exacerbations of asthma in primary care. Less than 50% of patients (irrespective of the type of therapy) had attained normal PEF levels after 16 days (Levy et al., 1996). There are few data for time intervals for follow-up and therefore each practice would need to agree its own policy. Perhaps further acute attacks and hospital readmissions could be reduced if patients were followed up more carefully than has been the case in the past. Subsequent monitoring by the practice needs to be arranged in such a way that defaulters are easily identified and invited to attend by one of the practice team dealing with asthma.

7

EDUCATION AND SELF-MANAGEMENT

INTRODUCTION

What is meant by education in asthma care? Most people would assume this to be about patient education, and indeed, a large part of this chapter is concerned with this. However, a review of the following case history reveals that parents, friends and health professionals all need some form of education in order to be of help.

Case history

MA is a 27-year-old female. She 'inherited' her asthma, by this she means that her father has had asthma all his life and she has had it for as long as she can remember. As a child, she would be given half of one of his tablets if her asthma was 'bad' and told that she would simply have to cope. As a teenager she was prescribed a salbutamol inhaler and nothing else. She would not tell her friends she had asthma – after all, her father always kept quiet about his. Her general practitioner colluded with her inappropriate behaviour by issuing repeat prescriptions without question. Her asthma is severe; at the age of 19 she had a respiratory arrest and since then she has had two admissions to intensive care. She is now in the care of a respiratory physician who she likes and respects immensely. She has a prescription for high-dose inhaled steroids, but takes these only at night. She is bright and lively. She is aware that the inhaled steroids are preventive in action, but worries about gaining weight if she uses them too much. Her boyfriend is bewildered by her asthma.

This case history poses a dramatic, but by no means unique, management problem. MA's beliefs about asthma, inculcated by her father's response to it, are currently too strong to utilise the excel-

lent information and guidance she has been given for self-management. She still believes she should 'get by' with the use of a salbutamol inhaler.

All health professionals will agree that patient involvement is a vital part of the management of any chronic condition, and asthma is a particularly good example of this. It is also probably fair to say that most doctors prefer dealing with the diagnosis and treatment rather than the educational aspects of a condition. This may explain why there is still a good deal of uncertainty and inconsistency in the ways in which patient education in asthma is delivered in primary care. This chapter will examine some of the accumulating evidence concerning the most effective ways of delivering patient education and how that makes an impact on self-management strategies for patients.

Other aspects covered in this chapter include education about asthma in schools and education of peers, relatives and friends. The education of those professionals who have to deal with asthma is covered in Chapter 9.

COMPLIANCE, ADHERENCE OR CONCORDANCE?

What exactly is patient education and what is its purpose? Is it really about ensuring that the patient has the opportunity to understand asthma and the reasons for taking treatment? One rather narrow justification from the health professional's viewpoint might be that education will improve patient 'compliance' with treatment. There is much evidence to suggest problems with compliance in chronic conditions. Studies using electronic recording devices incorporated in inhalers have suggested compliance levels well below 50%.

The *Oxford Dictionary* defines compliance as *"action implementing wishes or commands"*. Is it surprising that perhaps more than half of our patients do not like being told what to do and therefore do not do it? The term compliance is viewed by many as an unsatisfactory indicator of the relationship between doctor and patient in prescribing for chronic conditions. Adherence is an alternative term that implies the degree to which a patient sticks to the agreed dosage regimen for a treatment. More recently, concordance has been proposed as a preferable term (Mullen, 1997) indicating much more of a partnership between doctor and patient in the decision about management. This is particularly appropriate for chronic conditions such as asthma, where even joint signature of prescriptions between doctor and patient has been mooted (Collier and Hilton, 1998). Whatever term we use in considering patients' responses to prescribed treatment, it is clear that problems can arise at a number of points in the transactions between prescribers and users (see Table 7.1).

The overall strategy of patient education and self-management must be to optimise the use of prescribed treatment in a partnership between the health professional and the patient, so that misunderstandings between the parties or even deceptions, are kept to a minimum. Probably, the most important facet of establishing an effective partnership is to give the patients the opportunity to express their beliefs and anxieties regarding the condition and its treatments.

Primary
A complete unwillingness to adhere to certain prescribed treatments; may be overt or covert

Secondary
Irregular adherence to such treatments; may be conscious or unconscious

Tertiary
Willing but ineffective adherence, particularly in technical matters such as inhaler or injection technique; may be deliberate or accidental

In all cases, poor communication between medical staff and patients is likely to be at the root of the problem

---

Table 7.1 Levels of non-compliance

Source: Hilton SR (1992) Does patient education work? *British Journal of Hospital Medicine* **47** (6): 438-441. Reproduced with permisson of Mark Allen Publishing Ltd.

At its simplest, patient education consists of providing information to patients about the condition itself and the treatment approaches required. There are some basic rules for the effective passing on of information to patients in the consultation. These were described by Ley, a psychologist (Ley, 1976). He has produced suggestions which aim to improve the dissemination of medical information from doctors to patients. These were:

- give instructions and advice early on in the interview
- stress the importance of this advice
- use short words and short sentences
- arrange information into clear categories
- repeat advice
- give specific advice rather than general recommendations

It is highly unlikely that patients will be able to recall more than five items of information from one interview, and usually they will remember the first (primacy rule) and last things that are said.

These and other suggestions were incorporated into a booklet used by general practitioners in a study on improving communication in common illnesses. Following the introduction of the booklet to doctors, the results showed significantly improved recall by patients. However, there were no significant changes in mean reported patient comprehension, satisfaction or confidence. This indicates that providing information about a condition is perhaps not sufficient.

Knowledge
Few patients with asthma are truly well informed about their condition and many studies have confirmed this (Ellis and Friend, 1985; Partridge, 1986; Hilton et al., 1986). Undoubtedly, the position has improved in recent years following major initiatives in primary care and the enormous contribution made by the National Asthma Campaign in helping to raise the profile of asthma as a condition to the general population, and their provision of high quality patient information materials. The pharmaceutical industry has also made notable contributions to the field of patient information in asthma.

Attitudes and beliefs

Sibbald, in a study (1989) of patients' beliefs and attitudes to asthma, and their responses to a number of hypothetical situations, found that feelings of stigma and panic to acute asthma were more likely to be related to inappropriate self-management behaviours. This related particularly to a tendency to overuse bronchodilators rather than seek medical advice. Studies in Holland have suggested that the duration of hospitalisation for patients with acute asthma was more closely related to certain psychological features, such as stigma, anxiety or hostility, than to more objective measures of severity of asthma on admission.

Other psycho-social factors may be important in determining patients' responses to uncontrolled asthma, or their concordance with treatment in general. These include: depression and anxiety; shame, anger or stigmatisation because of asthma; and social isolation.

Studies of the effects of patient education

Evidence has already been cited to urge caution in dispensing information in an unsupported way. It is worth noting some of the studies that have pinpointed the pitfalls of patient education. Interest has turned to the benefits of educating asthma patients in groups rather than individually. One American study made such a comparison in a large controlled trial and the results showed group education to be superior (Wilson et al., 1993). Educational steps proposed at the end of this chapter arise from the evidence provided by studies in the following sections.

USA studies

The most conclusive study, carried out by Fireman and colleagues (1981), reported a controlled trial in asthmatic children aged 2 to 14 years. Children and their parents were given four hours of instruction in all aspects of asthma and its management, and were given regular support and follow-up. In the following year, there was a tenfold reduction in school absence and significantly fewer hospital attendances and acute attacks of asthma in the treatment group. In their controlled trial of health education for adult asthmatics, Maiman and colleagues (1979), using a complex intervention studied the effects of the type of person providing education. They found that a nurse, who was herself an asthmatic, was a significantly more effective communicator than an 'unaffected' nurse. This resulted in fewer emergency room visits. In New York, a large controlled trial was carried out on over 300 children from low income (Evans et al., 1987). Their intervention was a package of one hour programmes, for children and their parents, offered by health educators in English and Spanish. Overall effects of the intervention on morbidity, over one year, were disappointingly small, except in the sub-group with the most severe asthma. These studies, despite good resources, only showed convincing beneficial effects in patients with more severe asthma.

UK studies

There were no comparable studies in the United Kingdom before the 1980s. A controlled trial, carried out in general practice, set out to test the hypothesis that an improvement in asthma patients' knowledge would reduce morbidity (Hilton et al., 1986). A population of 339 asthma patients, recruited from 34 general practices in South London was assessed prior to an intervention in two of three groups, which included booklets, audio tapes and consultations for review of asthma knowledge. Reassessment took place after one year. In both groups, knowledge of asthma increased but neither group showed any improvement in self-management ability or asthma morbidity that differed significantly from changes in the control group. Thus, knowledge was improved but behaviour did not change and morbidity was not improved by the intervention.

A general practice study, in Nottingham, on 177 patients (Jenkinson et al., 1988) looked at the effects of two forms of specially prepared educational material – an audio tape and a booklet. This study compared the knowledge, attitudes, self-management and morbidity of the patients. Knowledge of drug usage was significantly increased for at least 12 months in the groups receiving either or both forms of education. Perception of disability caused by asthma fell (though not significantly) in all groups receiving the material, but there were no significant change in self-management or morbidity as a result of the interventions.

A general practice study was carried out in Scotland, where a review of patients' asthma by a research nurse was accompanied by a patient education programme (Crosby et al., 1989). Feedback from the review nurse was given to the GPs of the patients. After one year there were significant improvements in symptoms and peak expiratory flow readings compared with controls, and significantly less time missed from work in the most severely affected sub-group. Other studies have shown patient education to be effective in reducing short and medium-term morbidity, but only in the interested minority that responded to invitations to participate in the study (Yoon et al., 1993).

Self-management

Overall, 'pure' patient education approaches produced only modest effects on asthma morbidity, with most benefit occurring, not surprisingly, in those with more severe asthma. This is not necessarily helpful to general practices with large numbers of asthma patients on their lists - many of whom are mildly affected. There was evidence that behavioural approaches were more effective than the didactic informative styles of some earlier programmes (Mazzuca et al., 1992). The notion that patients should 'know what to do and when' became prominent. Experimentation and evaluation became more focused on self-management programmes which might have included elements of patient education, but which relied much more on providing decisions for adjusting medication in the light of deteriorating symptoms or lung function.

United Kingdom

In Southampton, a written self-management programme was evaluated in an open study of 30 moderately severe patients with asthma, attending an asthma outpatient clinic (Beasley et al., 1989). All patients had their lung function 'optimised' by treatment with inhaled steroids before starting the evaluation. The self-management plan was individ-

ualised for patients but the basic plan was standard. The crucial feature of the plan was the adjustment of treatment levels according to peak flow thresholds. Nearly half the patients felt sufficiently confident in using their plan to initiate oral steroid courses without consulting their doctors. In the six months following the introduction of the plans, there were significant reductions in: morbidity; the number of days off work; oral steroid use, plus significant improvements in lung function

Charlton and colleagues carried out important studies on the effects of introducing a nurse-run asthma clinic in a group practice in Aylsham, Norfolk (Charlton et al., 1991). Of the 8,000 patients in the practice, 5.2% were diagnosed as asthmatic. Around 55% of these were on preventive treatment and were invited to attend an asthma clinic. The nurse ran the clinic for around ten hours per week – a significant investment of time – and devised self management plans with the patients. Half were peak flow driven, and half were driven by symptom changes. After one year, there were significant reductions in the number of rescue courses of oral steroids, acute nebulisations, and GP consultations compared with the year prior to the introduction of the clinic. Of course, there were many more consultations with the nurse. The peak flow driven and symptoms only self-management plans were not significantly different to each other in their effects.

Jones carried out a randomised controlled trial on 72 general practice patients, attempting to replicate the work of Beasley and Holgate on hospital outpatients in 1989 (see above). Although there were some quality of life advantages for the intervention group, there were no significant differences in lung function, symptoms or treatment costs (Jones et al., 1995).

The GRASSIC study was a large and important collaborative project between hospitals and general practices in the Grampian region of Scotland, around Aberdeen (Grampian Asthma Study of Integrated Care, 1994). The study, a randomised controlled trial using 569 patients, evaluated a three step treatment plan amongst general practice asthma patients who were not already using peak flow meters at home (thereby excluding a large number of more severely affected patients). Those receiving self-management information were given an individually tailored three step plan, with instructions to commence oral corticosteroids at certain thresholds. The impact of the self-management plans were limited, conferring only modest benefits, such as less restriction of activities in those given a PEF meter, and receiving integrated care.

A number of studies from around the world have suggested that self-management plans are valuable and lead to reductions in morbidity.

Finland

Lahduenso compared self-management of asthma with usual follow-up in moderate to severe asthmatics – all were on at least moderate dosages of inhaled steroids (Lahdensuo et al., 1996). Although there were no objective differences in lung function between groups after one year, the need for emergency visits, time off work, rescue course of steroids and antibiotics were approximately halved in the intervention group compared to the control group. Quality of life scores were also more favourable in the intervention group.

New Zealand

D'Souza offered a 'credit card' self-management plan approach to 69 adults attending A&E with acute asthma (D'Souza et al., 1996). Brief, compact guidance was provided with symptoms on one side of the card and PEF readings on the reverse. Although numbers were small, and recruitment bias was likely, the results (in terms of reducing re-attendances at A&E) were impressive. Results from the trial prompted the National Asthma Campaign in the UK to produce similar materials for patients. The convenience of a miniaturised and simplified self-management plan is clearly attractive. They are undoubtedly helpful and popular for some patients, although a large-scale controlled evaluation of their effectiveness has not been carried out.

Spain

Ignacio-Garcia carried out a study on 70 patients which gave individualised instructions to patients regarding medication adjustment (Ignacio-Garcia et al., 1995). Over a six month period there were significant reductions in time lost from work, in exacerbations, and in hospital admissions compared with controls.

Canada

Bernard-Bonnin reported a meta-analysis of paediatric self-management programmes. Although 23 randomised controlled trials were identified from the literature as relevant, only 11 were considered sufficiently rigorous in their design to be included in the meta-analysis. The analysis indicated a non-significant effect-size on school absenteeism, acute attacks and emergency attendance at hospital (Bernard-Bonnin et al., 1995).

In reviewing these and other self-management studies, van der Palen and colleagues concluded that the picture is far from clear. They distinguished between a broader self-management approach, which includes greater understanding of prevention, environment modification, seeking help etc, from self-treatment where the focus is on adjustment of medication in response to changes in symptoms or PEF readings. For self-treatment, the evidence for self-efficacy is not particularly convincing (van der Palen et al., 1998).

Implications for the primary care team

Given such a range of results from differing environments around the world, what is the primary care team to make of this evidence when considering its own approach to patient self-management plans? General practice in the UK has benefited greatly from a pragmatic approach that recognises the differing needs of individuals. Many research studies are carried out under artificial conditions and are concerned with the 'efficacy' of an intervention (ie whether it 'works' under ideal conditions) rather than its effectiveness (how it performs under the constraints of day-to-day practice). Others, including more recent community-based studies, make every effort to root their evaluations in the realities of clinical practice. It must be said that such studies have yet to produce incontrovertible evidence for the benefits of self-treatment plans.

In the age of evidence-based medicine, it is ironic that those research studies which try most closely to match real practice find themselves too constrained by practicalities to be included as methodologically sound in systematic reviews. The tensions between pragmatic and explanatory trials are well recognised. Edwards and colleagues have argued for greater consideration to be given to those studies which may not reach the highest standards of rigour, but produce an important or consistent message (Edwards et al., 1998).

Thus, the studies in UK general practice from Charlton, GRASSIC, Jones and more recently from Dickinson (Dickinson et al., 1997) reveal a mixture of approaches and results. The GRAS-SIC study, and Jones and colleagues, applied the randomised controlled trial design as rigorously as possible. Both found themselves having to exclude those patients most likely to benefit from the intervention, in the former because of prior 'contamination', and in the latter because of recruitment difficulties. Both the Charlton and Dickinson studies showed impressive reductions in morbidity in the patients studied, but as uncontrolled experiments they were open to criticisms about their methodology; and in evidence-based practice their findings would be placed further down the hierarchy than GRASSIC and Jones.

Clearly, it is good practice to give patients high quality information, preferably written, about their condition and its causes and treatments. The level to which we should be pushing self-treatment plans, with detailed medication adjustments, is less clear. This is a matter which should be explored jointly by the patient and the health professionals concerned. If the patient has mild to moderate asthma and little interest in creating a self-treatment plan, the evidence suggests that the benefits (for all concerned) from imposing one, will be minimal. Patients with severe asthma or who are prone to troublesome exacerbations should be targeted for agreed self-management plans. Each case will, of course, be different. The following factors are likely to influence concordance between health professionals and patients and all should be considered when drawing up self-management plans:

- previous experience of asthma
- feelings of anger, denial, shame or stigma about having asthma
- social isolation
- concurrent anxiety and/or depression
- relevant lifestyle factors eg smoker, peer pressure in teenagers

PARENTS, RELATIVES AND FRIENDS

Parents form a special group. In childhood asthma they form the focus of patient education and carry out self-management on behalf of their child. Where parents also suffer from asthma it is common to find that they are much more assiduous in the care of the child's asthma than their own. Most parents are highly motivated and receptive to information and ideas about asthma. Problems tend to arise as the child grows as there is conflict over who should be in control of the asthma. This usually comes to a head during the teenage years, but may occur long before then. One of the commonest complaints received from young people is that the doctor continues to talk through them to the parent. Their natural reticence makes it difficult for them to intervene and change the flow of the consultation.

Relatives, friends and peers may be more peripheral to the day-to-day control of treatment, but their attitudes to the individual and to asthma in general may have a considerable impact. Many misconceptions about asthma continue to be held by members of the public, and it is known that many people with asthma feel stigmatised by their condition.

The corollary of this is that as much emphasis should be given to public awareness campaigns on asthma as should be given to individual patient education. The National Asthma Campaign has achieved a remarkable amount in this respect during the 1990s.

SCHOOLS

Schoolteachers, particularly in primary schools, carry a good deal of responsibility for the care of asthma. Most classes of average size will have at least two or three children with asthma and it is important that they should be given the best opportunities to function normally in the classroom, in the playground, and on the sports field. Until recent years, it seemed that there was worrying unfamiliarity with asthma in schools. Surveys in London (Bevis and Taylor, 1990) and Sussex (Storr et al., 1987) reported similar findings – poor knowledge of the mode of action of treatments, with the exception of salbutamol and a widespread uncertainty about correct actions to take during attacks. In many schools children's inhalers were locked into medicine cabinets, inaccessible during times of need. All teachers should be aware of the likely precipitants of asthma symptoms; basic facts about anti-asthma medication, including how to operate a chamber device; and how to respond if a child with asthma becomes acutely unwell.

In recent years, as a result of enormous efforts and initiatives by the major asthma charities, the National Asthma Campaign and the National Asthma and Respiratory Training Centre, the management of asthma in schools has been transformed in most parts of the UK. National Asthma Week initiatives, with provision of information packs by the former and excellent publications and training courses for school nurses by the latter, have raised the profile of asthma care in school and demolished outdated myths concerning access to inhalers. In many local initiatives, schools, parents and health professionals have produced school policies for asthma care.

The primary school is also an environment where undiagnosed asthma is likely to express itself and teachers who are aware of the frequency of the condition can play a part, in conjunction with school medical services and parents, in identifying new cases.

HEALTH PROFESSIONALS

As with the National Asthma Campaign and public awareness, the National Asthma and Respiratory Training Centre (now based in Warwick) has revolutionised the in-service training of primary care professionals in asthma management. The role of the asthma-trained nurse in organised care for asthma is discussed in detail in Chapter 9. A range of postgraduate and post-registration diplomas have been developed by the centre, some in conjunction with other institutions. Other smaller centres, in different parts of the country, have followed suit and the standards of care provided by health professionals in primary care have risen steadily as a consequence.

Specialist respiratory nurses in the hospital setting are also playing increasingly important roles in patient education, and some outreach schemes have had very favourable evaluations. Madge reported on a controlled trial involving an outreach paediatric nurse in Glasgow (Madge et al., 1997). Two hundred children aged two or more, who had been admitted to hospital with acute asthma, were randomised. The intervention group received a home management programme administered by the nurse and this was followed-up with information and telephone contact. Subsequent readmissions were reduced from 25% to 8% in the intervention group and there were also significant improvements in other morbidity indices compared with the control group.

With increasing importance of community-based primary care, the contributions of other health professionals such as pharmacists, physiotherapists and some complementary therapists, are also growing.

CONCLUSIONS

Two messages are crucial to a basis for effective education. They may be self-evident, but we make no apology for this. The first is that it is essential to discover, by letting patients express their wishes, what it is they want to know about asthma. If they are able to do this, then they may reveal their wishes, prejudices and beliefs about asthma.

The second is that all patients are individuals, with different needs, attitudes and beliefs. Hence, the standard educational package should not really exist. It is certainly a good idea to have a wide range of preferred times, leaflets, charts, booklets but it should be accepted that they will prove unacceptable to some patients. Information should be viewed as part of the much wider goal of involving patients in discussion about their asthma.

8

INHALER DEVICES

INTRODUCTION

The inhaled route is currently accepted as the most effective for asthma management. A hand-held inhaler device should be prescribed as a first choice wherever possible. Selection of the appropriate device for delivery of an asthma drug depends upon a number of factors. The clinical effect of an inhaled drug depends upon its potency and the amount delivered to the lungs, which in turn is influenced by the dose and particle size emitted from the inhaler device. Furthermore, the dose expelled from the orifice of the device influences the amount available to reach the lungs. The systemic effect (including side effects) of an inhaled drug is determined by the amount of active drug absorbed from the lung and the gut, coupled with the degree to which this is inactivated by the liver.

It may be difficult to decide which asthma patients (based on severity or age) will benefit from particular combinations of drug and inhaler device. While many characteristics of various drug-inhaler device combinations are known, there is often insufficient information to enable the clinician to select easily between them. Consequently, we must rely on the clinical outcome of prescribing and the results of subsequent alterations in dosage. It is beyond the scope of this book to describe all the devices in detail and we refer the reader to other excellent publications on different devices and drugs available (Pedersen, 1996; Barnes et al., 1997); and also to the *Monthly Index of Medical Specialities* – MIMS – supplied to every doctor in the UK. This chapter highlights some of the important clinical and practical issues related to asthma inhaler devices.

ARE INHALER DEVICES EQUIVALENT?

This is a difficult question to answer. How is equivalence assessed? Are we comparing drugs, devices or the combinations of both? Asthma drugs are compared in the laboratory, on machines or experimental animals, through clinical trials on normal or asthmatic subjects. A machine or test rig with consistent characteristics may facilitate fair comparisons of various characteristics between different drug/device combinations. These include inspiratory flow required to deliver the drug from the orifice of the device, the amount delivered and the range of drug particle sizes. However, people with asthma respond differently to combinations of drugs and devices; this may vary in individuals depending on their asthma severity at the time. Drug trials are expensive and often funded by the manufacturer of one particular device. As a result, there are few comparative trials which enable a clinician to make a clear choice between different drug/device combinations. Research has clarified that people with asthma may benefit from a number of combinations, with variability within individuals over time. Hence, clinicians should not be too rigid in their choice of asthma device and should be prepared to try different combinations of prescription according to the clinical response.

CFCs (CHLOROFLUROCARBONS) AND HFAs (HYDROFLUOROALKANES)

The worldwide acceptance that CFCs (chlorofluorocarbons) are harmful to the atmosphere has resulted in the identification and development of alternative propellants, HFAs (hydrofluoroalkanes) for delivering drugs via pressurised metered

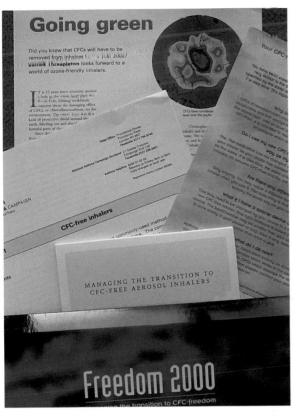

Figure 8.1 CFC to CFC-Free changeover: A selection of leaflets from the NAC and pharmaceutical industry (3M Pharmaceuticals and Allen and Hanburys)

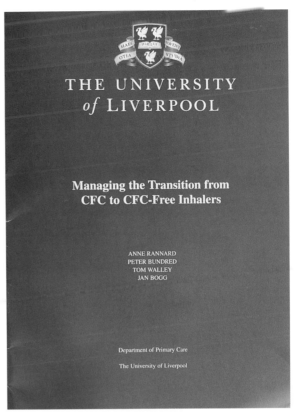

Figure 8.2 CFC to CFC-Free changeover: a helpful, informative publication from the University of Liverpool's Department of Primary Care

dose inhalers (pMDIs). At the time of writing, two drugs are available in the UK via pMDIs that use HFAs; salbutamol (Airomir) and beclomethasone dipropionate (QVAR) both made by 3M Health Care; and salbutamol (Ventolin Evohaler, Glaxo Wellcome) is currently available in Scotland and Northern Ireland. Other pharmaceutical companies have developed CFC-free products; beclomethasone pMDI (Baker Norton) which is currently available in Ireland.

The introduction of these new devices requires an organised transition program in primary and secondary care. QVAR (3M Beclomethasone dipropionate) has been granted a UK prescription licence at half the dose of CFC-beclomethasone; generic prescriptions may lead to confusion and patients may not administer the dose intended by their doctor. Therefore, it is safer to prescribe this drug by brand name. Drugs delivered via the HFA devices taste different, they hit the back of the

throat with less force and there is no 'cold freon' effect (cold sensation at the back of the throat). These differences should be explained to patients.

Figures 8.1 and 8.2 illustrate some of the leaflets and documentation available to assist clinicians in the changeover to CFC-free inhalers.

CHOOSING AN INHALER DEVICE

Pedersen (1996) summarised the most important questions to consider when prescribing an inhaler (see Table 8.1). His review paper discussed many of the difficulties in interpreting studies on asthma devices and applying the results to clinical practice.

Correct usage is important, although 'correct' may be difficult to define. For example, the speed at which someone inhales a drug through an inhaler will determine whether the drug reaches the lungs; or if a child blows into a Turbohaler before inhaling, the dose delivered to the orifice of the device may reduce. So health professionals need to be aware of the characteristics of different devices (and therefore the inhalation methods patients need to use) in order to deliver the optimum amount of respirable drug particles to the lungs (generally accepted as particles below five microns). Health professionals prescribe pMDIs more frequently than other devices and this is usually related to their low cost and to patient preference. However, these are the most difficult devices to teach and to use. Furthermore, patients tend to forget the correct technique soon after initial demonstration, so this needs to be reinforced regularly.

The approach to selecting inhaled medication is to establish what would be suitable for the patient's age and ability, firstly by demonstrating, and then testing the patient's technique. This task is time consuming but vital to successful treatment. Clearly, appointments in a dedicated asthma clinic facilitate this. Various samples of the different devices enable the patient to test their ability and choose a device. A drug suitable for the chosen device is then prescribed.

The In-check inhaler assessment kit (see Figure 8.3) does offer clinicians some assistance in choosing which device to prescribe initially for a patient. The kit comprises of a peak inspiratory flow meter and a number of variable resistance adapters (designed to mimic some of the inhaler devices) which fit between the device and the mouthpiece. Thus, the meter is able to assess the inspiratory flow rate generated by a patient under similar circumstances to those encountered when using the actual device.

- Which inhaler is the simplest and easiest to use according to the patient's age and ability?
- Which inhaler delivers the highest fraction of the dose of the particular drug required, to the intrapulmonary airways?
- Which inhaler has the best clinical effect relative to the systemic effect (the therapeutic ratio)?
- Which inhaler does the patient prefer?

Table 8.1 Selecting an inhaler

Source: Pedersen, 1996

If a child is able to generate an inspiratory flow of around 30L/min it would be appropriate to prescribe an Autohaler or an Easi-breathe inhaler because this is the optimum flow rate for drug delivery from these devices. Optimum delivery of the dose through a Turbohaler requires a minimum of 30L/min and ideally 60L/min (Borgstrom and Newman, 1993) inspiratory flow. The delivery of a drug from the Accuhaler is fairly consistent across the inspiratory flow range from 30 to 90L/min (Malton et al., 1996; Nielsen et al., 1998).

Confusion may occur with children who are expected to blow into a peak flow meter when they are still having difficulties learning to suck. We would suggest concentrating first upon the inhaler technique.

The Haleraid (see Figure 8.4) is useful for arthritic patients and can be used together with a Volumatic. It is a device that fits the Allen and Hanburys metered dose inhalers and enables people with arthritis or weak joints to use them. This is for sale by retail pharmacists in the UK.

Where is the drug delivered?

During initiation, the drug is deposited in the inhaler device, the oropharynx and the lungs. A further fraction is exhaled without reaching the lungs. In the case of most inhaled drugs, the proportion deposited in the mouth determines the level of potential adverse systemic effect. The CFC-containing pMDIs deliver about 80% of the drug to the oropharynx and only about 10% reaches the airways (Pedersen, 1996). This is not the case with the newer HFA driven pMDIs where drug deposition in the lungs is higher. Large volume spacers are used in conjunction with pMDIs in order to reduce the amount of drug deposited in the mouth.

TYPES OF INHALER DEVICE

There are four types of hand-held inhaler devices for treating asthma and COPD (see box); the other method for delivering inhaled drugs is via a nebuliser, either with a compressor or driven directly by high flow oxygen. While some drugs are available via different devices, their therapeutic effect (ratio

Types of inhaler device

1. Pressurised Metered Dose Inhalers (pMDIs)
Press and breath
  pMDIs (most companies)

  Breath actuated
  Autohaler (3M Health Care)
  Easi-Breathe (Baker Norton, Glaxo Wellcome)

2. Dry powder devices (Breath operated)
  Accuhaler (Allen & Hanbury's)
  Aerohaler (3M)
  Clickhaler (ML Laboratories)
  Diskhaler (Allen & Hanburys)
  Foradil Inhaler (Ciba Geigy)
  Rotahaler (Allen & Hanburys)
  Spinhaler (Fisons, RPR)
  Turbohaler (Astra)

3. Devices with integral spacers
  Integra (Allen & Hanbury's)
  Spacehaler (Evans)
  Syncroner (Fisons, RPR)
  Optimiser (with Easibreathe)

4. Spacers
  Small volume
  Aerochamber (3M Health Care)
  Babyhaler (3M Health Care)

  Large volume (used together with pMDIs)
  Fisonair (Fisons, RPR)
  Nebuhaler (Astra)
  Volumatic (Allen & Hanburys)

  Nebulisers
  Jet (most companies)
  Advanced
    Sidestream (Medic-aid)
    Ventstream (Medic-aid)
    Pari Plus (Pari)
  Adaptive
    Halolite (Medic-aid)

PARTICULAR CHARACTERISTICS AND USEFUL TIPS WHEN PRESCRIBING INHALER DEVICES

General advice for all patients: mouth rinse after use (eg use before brushing teeth).

1. pMDIs

These devices are difficult to use correctly and consistently. However, they are significantly cheaper than other types, and patients with satisfactory inhaler technique should be prescribed them, particularly where they prefer them! Beta-2 agonist bronchodilators are easily delivered to patients in emergencies with a pMDI (using a large volume spacer or polystyrene coffee cup). It may be difficult to determine whether a CFC inhaler is empty or not, although patients often learn to judge this well. In the case of HFA pMDI devices, these stop functioning when they are empty.

Advantages of HFA (CFC-free inhalers)

- the dose of drug delivered to the mouth is more consistent
- the device only needs to be shaken once every two weeks
- less drug is deposited in the mouth
- no cold-freon effect (The CFC inhalers result in a cold sensation at the back of the throat. Some patients get a fright when this happens; they stop inhaling and withdraw the inhaler from their mouth, resulting in inadequate inhalation)
- when the device is empty it stops functioning

While the CFC-free pMDIs may not be shaken as frequently as their CFC counterparts, it is often necessary to actuate these devices (prime them) once or twice when new or if they have not been used for a long while.

2. Breath actuated pMDIs

These devices eliminate the need for co-ordination between pressing and breathing; after priming the device (clicking a lever or removing the cap) all the patient needs to do is breathe in and hold breath for ten seconds.

of clinical to systemic effect) may vary. For example, budesonide delivered by a Turbohaler is twice as effective as through a pMDI (Borgstrom et al., 1996; Agertoft and Pedersen, 1994).

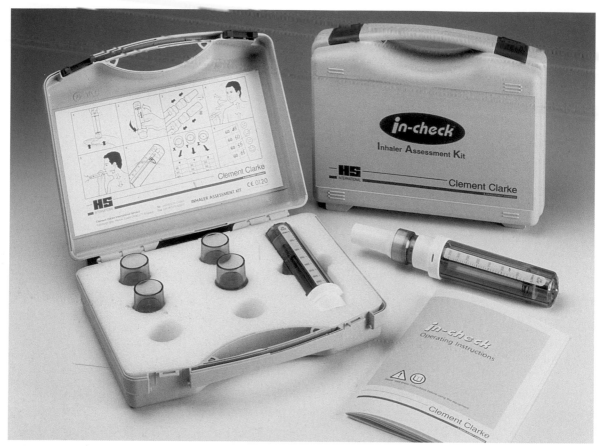

Figure 8.3 The In-check inhaler assessment kit

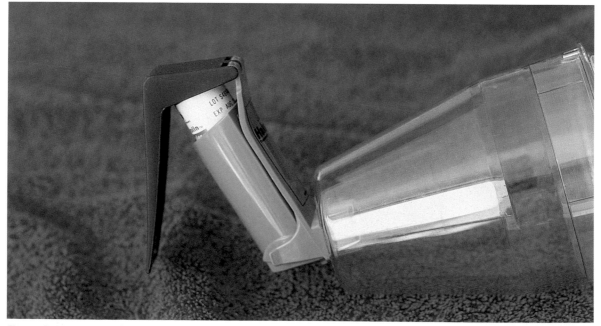

Figure 8.4 The Haleraid

3. Dry powder inhaler devices (DPIs)

These devices are breath actuated and require a degree of inspiratory flow generated by the patient. The In-check (see above) may be helpful in determining whether a patient is able to use a device and then which to choose. This is important with devices that require a certain inspiratory flow to disperse the drug into respirable particles. In the example quoted above, the Turbohaler requires at least 30L/min and optimally 60L/min to operate correctly.

4. Spacers

Spacers reduce the amount of drug deposited in the mouth, and subsequently entering the GI tract. Drug delivery to the lungs may be reduced by drug deposition within the spacer before it reaches the mouthpiece. This occurs as a result of gravity, speed of the impaction and 'static'. The newer CFC-free inhalers have a slower rate of delivery, resulting in less impaction (potentially more of the drug available for inhalation) within the spacer. Static electricity attracts deposition of drug on the surface of large volume spacer devices. A simple test can be used to determine whether there is significant static within a spacer. Hold a small piece of tissue paper next to a spacer: if the tissue sticks, static is present and the spacer needs to be rinsed. Static is removed (temporarily) by washing the spacer with soapy water (without rinsing it) and then drying it in air (not wiping). This needs to be done frequently, probably every week or two (O'Callaghan and Barry, 1997). Alternatively, the spacer may be primed (to reduce static) by expelling 10 to 15 puffs of bronchodilators within. This latter method is clearly wasteful and we only advocate its use in emergencies, where a patient needs high doses of bronchodilators through a brand new spacer.

Two methods are advocated for using spacers:

- single breath and breath holding
- continuous tidal breathing; (between 5 and 10 breaths depending on the size of the spacer and the size of the patient)

Spacers are useful in emergencies. It is widely accepted that spacers can be used as alternatives to nebulisers for acute asthma and for treating COPD. However, oxygen-driven nebulised beta-2 bronchodilators remain the best option for treatment of acute severe asthma. Smaller spacers need fewer breaths to empty and are therefore better for young children.

When using a spacer with a mask attached to deliver inhaled topical steroids in children, there is a risk of adverse effects from drug deposited on the face and it is important to remember to wash the face afterwards.

5. Nebulisers

Many people confuse the nebuliser with the compressor. The latter is used to deliver air at a flow rate high enough to create a mist in the nebuliser. A nebuliser is a small plastic device that converts the liquid drug into a fine mist when gas (air or oxygen) is driven through its narrowed inlet. A negative pressure is created, which draws liquid from the chamber and converts it into a fine mist (Bellamy and Ed Levy, 1998).

When delivering a drug by the nebulised route, mouthpieces should be used in preference to masks where possible. The mouthpiece results in less wastage and less drug deposition on the face. Nebulisers, mouthpieces, masks and tubing are licensed for single usage and should be discarded after use. They may not be prescribed on the NHS (FP10) and it is more cost-effective for general practitioners to use spacers and pMDIs wherever possible. Individual patients (eg with COPD or cystic fibrosis) may use these devices for about three months with appropriate attention to cleaning advice.

Many asthmatics experiencing nebuliser treatment for the first time, during an acute attack, view this treatment as special, almost magical. They will often ask their general practitioner about having one at home, to deal with any problems. However, patients may not understand that hospitals use oxygen to drive their nebulisers, while those used at home or in GP surgeries are driven by air compressors. We would urge health professionals to consider these requests very carefully. There are risks associated with air-driven nebulisers for acute asthma, in particular the resultant ventilation perfusion inequality that may dramatically reduce the arterial oxygen saturation. What this means is that the blood flow to the lungs may predominate in areas which are short of oxygen. As a result the level of oxygen carried in the arterial blood (the oxygen saturation of the haemoglobin) may be reduced. Secondly, patients may be lulled into a false sense of security and delay seeking assistance in the event of an attack.

The nebuliser is simply a device that delivers, in large doses, a drug the patient is probably taking already. There are two types, jet and ultrasonic. Jet nebulisers seem to be the more popular in terms of use, whilst ultrasonic types provide quieter but more expensive alternatives. In the jet type, a source of pressurised gas (usually a small electric compressor, alternatively a high flow air or oxygen cylinder, or a foot pump) 'sucks' the nebuliser solution up from a small chamber in the way described above. Ultrasonic nebulisers utilise a vibrating crystal, which sends a series of waves through the nebuliser solution, causing tiny particles to break off and form a mist.

Advantages and disadvantages of nebulisers

An easily inhaled mist, containing a high dose of drug, without the need for someone to administer the drug during the whole process, makes the nebuliser the simplest means of prescribing a bronchodilator during acute asthma. However, there is considerable debate regarding the efficiency of the method. Simple jet nebulisers deliver fairly large particles (too large for respiration) and there is a lot of wastage (see the GPIAG factsheet, Bellamy and Ed Levy, 1998 and Chapter 6 for more details). In between attacks any advantage of nebulisers over hand-held devices is less marked, since good technique with other devices enables sufficient drug to reach smaller airways. In anxious, hyperventilating asthmatic patients, the nebuliser may provide great reassurance and help to restore normal breathing.

Nebulisers are noisy, expensive and relatively cumbersome. Patients requiring regular nebulisations are more restricted in their activities than those carrying small inhaler devices in the pocket or handbag.

When to use nebulisers

• In the surgery and in the patient's home in emergencies

This is generally reserved for high dose administration of bronchodilators (salbutamol or terbutaline) during acute episodes. Whenever possible measure peak expiratory flow (PEF) and oxygen saturation before, (Levy, 1998) and regularly afterwards (see Chapter 6). Ipatropium bromide may have a useful additive effect if included with the bronchodilator, particularly in older patients. Bearing in mind that nebulised beta-2 agonist bronchodilators only clears bronchospasm and has minimal effects on the underlying congestion and hyperreactivity, other treatment will usually be required. Oral or inhaled topical corticosteroids are the only drugs that can treat this acute congestion effectively.

• Domiciliary nebulisers for patients

For most patients there are a range of alternative devices and treatment strategies. Regular preventive treatment, if necessary high dose preventive drugs via spacer devices, should be considered before recommending nebulisers for use at home.

There are two main groups of patients for which regular home use of a nebuliser are indicated:

1. The more severely affected preschool children who need nebulised preventive treatment (eg budesonide), because they cannot use other devices.
2. Older patients with severe chronic airflow obstruction who require regular high-dose bronchodilator treatment.

This form of drug delivery should only be prescribed after an initial home trial lasting three weeks, with peak flow monitoring (and spirometry if appropriate) and only after other methods of drug administration have been explored. Supervision should include evaluation of peak flow readings, monitoring of prescriptions and biannual servicing of the compressor.

The nebuliser is an efficient and sometimes dramatically successful means of delivering drug treatment for asthma. Given successful cooperation between doctor and patient, using agreed management plans and peak flow meters wherever possible, we believe nebulisers can be used successfully in the community, without mandatory referral to a specialist. However, provision of a nebuliser to a patient is not a substitute for careful explanation and instruction, and the general practitioner must be prepared to take the necessary time for this.

Problems with inhaled medication

Hoarseness and voice problems are the main problems encountered by some patients using inhaled drugs (particularly topical steroids). This may be due to local irritation resulting from the jet effect of the speed of delivery or oral thrush. These effects may be prevented by rinsing the mouth out after using inhalers, eating live natural yogurt or alternatively, one of the large spacer devices may be of help especially if high doses of inhaled topical steroids are being used.

Peak flow meters

There is a variety of peak flow meters available in the UK. These include the Wright's, the MiniWright's, the Vitallograph and the Pocket peak flow meters. The latter three are all cheap, light and suitable for the doctor's bag as well as home peak flow monitoring by patients. The Peak Flow Whistle is an alternative device that may be used in young children. A study in 101 children aged 3 to 12 years found that this device performed similarly to the Standard Wright Meter (Tsanakas et al., 1986). Clement Clarke International have also developed a 'Windmill device' to enable young children to learn how to use the peak flow meter in a consistent and reproducible fashion.

While the three types of PEF meter available on NHS prescription are reliable, their readings are not directly comparable; individual patients should use the same meter, whether for home or surgery monitoring. It follows that people with asthma should be prescribed their own meter and be encouraged to bring this to the surgery when consulting. Furthermore, it is important to understand that the scales used on these meters, in the UK, are not linearly related to the gold standard for measuring airflow ie a pneumotachograph. In practice, this results in over-reading in the lower PEF ranges and under-reading in the upper ranges (Miller and Levy, 1997). In other words, in a patient who normally produces a PEF around 300L/Min the PEF meter may produce an overestimated reading, resulting in a false sense of security for the health professional. Although this probably will not be clinically significant, it is worth remembering if someone in this category presents with symptoms of uncontrolled asthma and a normal PEF reading. Variability of a number of PEF readings is far more valuable as a clinical measurement than a single isolated reading.

9

ORGANISATION OF ASTHMA CARE

INTRODUCTION

Since the late 1980s considerable advances have occurred in the organisation of asthma care in the UK. This may be attributed to several factors:

- the changes to the General Practitioners' Contract in 1990
- the introduction of the Chronic Disease Management Programme in 1993
- the publication of National (British Thoracic Society et al) Asthma Guidelines (revised 1997)
- the availability of assessed and accredited asthma training for health professionals

It is difficult to quantify the impact of these changes individually, but emerging evidence supports their combined success (Pearson and Barnes 1987, Charlton et al., 1991, Neville et al., 1996).

As a result of the 1990 Health Promotion Regulations, and the subsequent Chronic Disease Management Programme, many asthma clinics were set up. It is important to appreciate that holding an asthma clinic is not the only way to organise good asthma care (Staples EB, 1991). A survey by the National Asthma Task Force (Barnes and Partridge 1993) showed that over 70% of practices with five or more partners ran an exclusive clinic for patients with asthma, whereas only 32% of single-handed general practitioners did so. However, the aim of this chapter is to examine some of the essentials needed to hold an asthma clinic and/or provide organised care, whether you are based in a single-handed inner-city practice or a large partnership in rural England.

ASTHMA CLINICS AND PRACTICE PROTOCOL

Where to start...

A small working group (perhaps only 2 to 3 people) within the primary health care team may formulate the practice protocol for management.

This should be circulated to the rest of the practice for comment, and be supported by them. The ideal members for this group would be a GP interested in asthma, a trained practice asthma nurse or a practice manager. The clear roles and responsibilities of members of the practice team in the organisation of asthma care should become apparent once the protocol has been formulated (eg recalling patients, targeting at risk patients etc).

The asthma register

The asthma register is the foundation stone on which to organise asthma care within the practice. It will identify the level of diagnosis, form part of the recall and review system and be an essential part of the audit process. Wherever possible, the register should include patients who are symptomatic but not taking treatment (for whatever reason) in addition to those patients currently receiving treatments. It should *not* include those people whose asthma symptoms have been in remission for more than an agreed length of time (usually 12 months) – see below.

If you are starting a register from scratch, firstly refer to the repeat prescriptions. These can be tagged on the computer system. This will also, however, identify those who are receiving bronchodilators and/or corticosteroids for other conditions – such as chronic obstructive pulmonary disease (COPD). Clearly it is preferable for the practice computer to have a system for tagging patients with a defined disease and pulling off those with the label 'asthma'. If by doing this, the number of asthma patients appears disproportionately low compared to national averages (approximately 140 asthma patients per 2,000 patients), you will also need some form of manual note search to build up your register. This can be a lengthy and ongoing process.

The computer system is the easiest way to maintain the register, although card systems can be used effectively. Maintaining and updating the register is an essential part of the provision of preventive asthma care. It is important for all newly diagnosed patients, as well as existing asthmatics who have not been included in the initial process, to be continually added to the asthma register. Some patients who are labelled 'asthma' may not be currently taking prescribed treatment and it may therefore be advisable to have a 'current (active) register' and 'in remission (non-active)' register. Decide a policy for the latter, so patients in remission are not forgotten about.

How often should asthma clinics be run?

This is dependent on the size of the asthma register and the availability of trained staff. You may decide to include the asthma patients in general chronic disease management or health promotion clinics; this may help to attract potential non-attenders. In order to accommodate various lifestyles it is helpful to offer a varied and accessible service. It may even be necessary to run several special asthma clinics each week.

Initial assessment in the asthma clinic

The initial assessment of a patient who is newly diagnosed, or is attending the clinic for the first time, may take between 30 and 45 minutes. It is therefore important to allow adequate time. Your practice protocol should specify the standard criteria which will be included within this assessment.

The following points should be included:
- current and past history
  - previous medical history
  - previous asthma history
  - previous asthma medication
  - current asthma medication (specify device and dose)
  - concurrent medication for other complaints (noting any NSAIDs, aspirin, beta-blockers)
- height, weight, peak flow predicted and actual, or spirometry if available
- inhaler device technique
- symptoms day, night exercise (preferably using a symptom scoring method)
- trigger factors and allergies
- occupational history

- smoking history (past, current or passive) - if current, ask about the number of cigarettes per day
- initial education about asthma and medication, including patient's own beliefs and attitudes
- diagnostic tests (select most appropriate)
  - exercise test
  - reversibility test
  - steroid trial
  - home peak flow and symptom monitoring for two weeks

Patient review in the asthma clinic

The frequency of review will be dependent on the severity of the patient's asthma, the patient's understanding and requirement for information about asthma and their ability to 'self-manage' their asthma.

Patients on high dose inhaled steroids should be reviewed every 3 to 6 months in order to assess whether their treatment can be reduced in line with the British Asthma Guidelines. All asthma patients receiving treatment should be reviewed annually. Other at risk patients (discussed later in the chapter) will need to be reviewed more frequently, as required.

The review session can be completed within 10 to 15 minutes if the session is well structured. Agree within the practice protocol the 'must be done' and the 'good to do if time is available'.

The following points should be included:
- enquire about and record symptoms and quality of life (symptom scoring is the easiest way to record and measure)
- enquire about and record medication dosage prescribed check and record peak expiratory flow or spirometry - note technique
- check and record inhaler technique; re-instruct if necessary
- enquire about compliance (discuss with patient and check computer repeat prescriptions)
- provide asthma education check and record a child's height using an accurate and consistent method make a follow-up appointment
- check repeat prescription status and update if necessary
- discuss and devise a self-management plan where appropriate

Targeting patients appropriately

In order to use the asthma clinic effectively and to ensure that the process of organised care within the practice is maximised, it is important to target patients appropriately. Patients who ought to be seen in the clinic as a priority are patients who are, or have been:

- newly diagnosed
- high users of short-acting beta agonists (one short acting reliever inhaler per month or more)
- recently admitted to hospital or attended A&E
- recently nebulised
- recently required a course of oral steroids
- high dose of inhaled steroids which may be able to be reduced
- children about to attend school for the first time

Patient referral

A referral policy between the doctors and the asthma nurse needs to be determined. Additionally a policy for referral to secondary care needs to be established (the British Asthma Guidelines give advice on hospital referral – see Chapter 5).

Referral within general practice may mean the doctor or the asthma nurse asking the patient to make a separate appointment with either the doctor or nurse, both the doctor and nurse seeing the patient together, or jointly discussing the patient's case history and management.

For referral within the practice a GPs in Asthma Group workshop publication made the following recommendations:

Doctor to nurse (either by formal appointment or informal discussion)

- patients should be referred by the doctor to the nurse-run asthma clinic
- there should be a doctor who can be called upon if the nurse is at all concerned about the patient
- there should be a system for reviewing the patients or their records jointly by the referring doctor and the nurse

Nurse to doctor (either by formal appointment or informal discussion)

- treatment is failing, ie the patient complains of symptoms which are not responding to treatment or the presence of exercise-induced or night-time symptoms
- the patient has had a recent severe asthma attack
- there is a need to introduce a short course of oral steroids
- the nurse is worried or lacks confidence about any aspect of the patient's management
- the patient does not seem to be receptive to the nurse's advice or management
- the patient's lung function and/or symptom score deteriorate below agreed levels
- there are side effects to drugs
- the patient presents to the nurse with symptoms unrelated to asthma

Treatment protocols

The practice treatment protocol needs to include drugs, devices, prescription and nebuliser policy as follows:

Drugs and devices

The British Asthma Guidelines position drugs and their dosages. It is advisable to work either within these or locally adapted guidelines to ensure consistency of approach within the practice.

There is now a plethora of inhaler devices. The advantage of this is that they offer a wide range of choice from which the health professional and patient can select. The disadvantage is that there are a large number of drugs and doses and devices to remember and advise patients about. Inevitably, patients will be established on a wide selection of devices. If they are well controlled, you may well decide to keep them on their existing device. However, you may wish to consider a more limited selection for new patients based on criteria such as: ease of use, ease of teaching, clinical data and cost.

It is advisable that if changing a patient's drug, drug dosage or device that they are monitored for success or failure by the patient completing a peak expiratory flow and symptom diary.

Prescriptions

All practices will have a repeat prescribing policy. With asthma, this needs to include:

- how patients obtain a repeat prescription
- the length of time the repeat prescriptions should run (time or quantity limited) before review
- updating the prescription on the computer at each asthma review
- the process for an emergency asthma prescription
- whether the asthma nurse can prepare the prescription for signature
- how the prescriptions should be worded and categorised on the computer (eg generically or by brand for drug and device)

With the advent of chlorofluorocarbon (CFC) free formulations, where different products deliver different amounts of drug to the lung, particular care is required to ensure that the patient continues to receive an equivalent dose from the prescribed inhaler.

Nebulisers

Nebulisers are invaluable for the delivery of high doses of bronchodilator to the lungs, but they are not without risks or problems. Ideally, oxygen should be administered with the nebulised bronchodilator. If faced with a choice between an air-driven nebuliser and a spacer, the latter is probably the best. It is desirable to have a policy that covers aspects of how the nebuliser is used: within the practice; during emergency call outs; and on loan to patients. Care and maintenance of the nebuliser is essential, and should also be included within the protocol. Guidelines for nebuliser use have been produced by the British Thoracic Society.

An essential part of delivering nebulised treatment is an assessment of the patient's peak expiratory flow before and after treatment. One study showed that general practitioners often failed to carry out this routine procedure (McKinley and Steele, 1995). Thus, a peak flow meter should be kept with each nebuliser within the practice and for emergency call-outs. In addition, a notebook which logs and records patients who have been nebulised is needed for follow-up and audit. All patients who have been nebulised should be followed-up within 12 hours.

The practice nebulisers should be regularly maintained. Tubing and nebuliser drug chambers, mouth pieces and masks should be cleaned and replaced according to the manufacturers guidelines. Where possible, patients should always use a mouthpiece.

Domicilary nebuliser loan should generally be avoided for the acute asthma patient as this can give the wrong message. They may conclude that the nebuliser is the only effective way to deliver treatment and may become over reliant on it and not seek help (Laroche et al., 1985). There is evidence to show that short-acting beta agonist delivered by metered dose inhaler via a large volume spacer is as effective as a nebuliser (Blake et al., 1992) (see also Chapters 6 and 8).

Auditing the asthma clinic

Audit is also discussed in Chapter 10. As part of routine organised care within the Chronic Disease Management Programme, practices are required to audit asthma care. Regardless of regulations it is advisable for the practice to develop a comprehensive audit system for its own benefit. Audit, conducted thoroughly, helps to ensure effectiveness of the care provided and to identify areas for improvement.

It is valuable to audit both process and outcomes. When auditing process you may wish to include the percentage of patients:

- seen
- on prophylaxis
- with a self-management plan (define what the practice means by this)
- whose inhaler technique has been checked

When auditing outcomes consider the number of patients requiring:

- hospital admissions
- emergency nebulisations
- an emergency call-out
- an emergency oral steroid course

The Tayside system is a simple rubber stamp, developed by a group of GPs in the Tayside area of Scotland. It uses a simple symptom scoring system that can be used routinely by everyone in the practice (see Chapter 5).

You will also be able to assess:

• night symptom scores
• daytime symptom scores
• exercise symptom scores
• time off work or school

Care within routine practice surgeries

For certain types of patients, or in some practices, a formal asthma clinic may not be appropriate. Nevertheless it remains essential that the care provided is organised and not randomly provided for the acute situation, as was the case in the past.

Even when asthma patients are seen within the normal surgery appointments the following aspects of care still apply:

• practice asthma protocol
• asthma register
• extended initial assessment appointments
• regularly recall and review of patients
• targeting of 'at risk' patients
• audit of care

USE OF SELF-MANAGEMENT PLANS

The term 'self-management plan' has come into wide usage in the field of asthma care. A patient self-management plan can vary from simple advice about when to make an appointment to visit the asthma clinic, to complex peak flow and symptom recording and treatment adjustment.

The subject is complex as it involves patient understanding and attitude to their condition and consequently compliance. Additionally, self-management is dependent on the verbal or written advice the health professional gives to the patient. Within this chapter the focus will be on advice given to patients, rather than the complexities of patient compliance psychology.

The aim of patient education should be that, at least to some degree, the asthma patient can manage their own disease. Numerous studies of the effects of education and patient self-management have been carried out and these have been reviewed in Chapter 7.

A feature of many of these studies is that successful self-management is achieved when the plans are individualised to the patient. It is important that the information given is simple and the patient is advised about what to do and when. The plan is better retained and adhered to by the patient if the information is written down.

RECORD KEEPING SYSTEMS

There are many ways to record information about the asthma patient. It is often desirable to use a combination of methods. Whatever system is adopted, the aim should be for uniformity throughout the practice, with all agreeing on the essential information to be recorded, and where. This helps continuity of patient care, communication and referral between GP partners and communication to and from the asthma clinic; it also facilitates audit. The current options are:

1. Computer records:

These vary greatly according to the system. Often they do not allow customisation to the practice and may not include all the information that you would like to record. It may be possible for you to use your own template and it is worth consulting your computer system provider. If using this system it is also valuable to have the ability to 'tag' information in order to audit and collate information

2. Patient notes

3. Tayside stamp (see page 42)

4. Asthma record card (available from the National Asthma and Respiratory Training Centre):

This card is designed to fit into the patient's notes. It covers the initial assessment and is a useful prompt. It also has space for routine follow-up information.

The method you decide to use should fit in with your existing systems and must be acceptable to all those within the practice.

ORGANISING FOLLOW-UP AND TARGETING THOSE AT RISK

Follow-up

All patients receiving asthma medication should be routinely reviewed at least once a year. This can be done effectively by using the asthma register or the repeat prescription system. A simple card file with the months of the year can be used. A card with patient names for review can be slotted into each month and letters sent out. One option is to include a two-week peak flow and/or symptom diary for the patient to complete in the fortnight leading up to the appointment. This may provide very useful information. Once the patient has been seen, their card can be allocated to another review month ie 3, 6, 9 or 12 months ahead.

Letters or cards should be sent to patients who do not attend for their scheduled review. These may be simple reminders that they are due to be seen, or might include an appointment date and time. Even if the appointment time has to be rearranged to suit the patient, this latter approach may be more effective.

Targeting those at risk

All asthma patients are theoretically 'at risk' of a life threatening attack. However, it is important to establish, within your practice protocol, which asthma patients should be targeted for special attention. Patients who are most vulnerable include those who are or have been:

- newly diagnosed
- high users of short-acting beta agonists (one short-acting reliever inhaler per month or more)
- recently admitted to hospital or attended A&E
- recently nebulised
- recently treated with a course of oral steroids taking more than three types of asthma medication
- depressed, anxious or suffering from psycho-logical problems

Patients who have been admitted to hospital or attended A&E should, according to the British Asthma Guidelines, be followed up within one week. Those who have been nebulised with high dose short-acting bronchodilators should be reviewed by the doctor, or asthma trained nurse, within 24 hours.

WHAT ABOUT NON-ATTENDERS?

In order to reduce the inevitable problem of non-attenders to asthma clinics some simple steps can be taken.

1. Aim to provide a varied service – daytime sessions for elderly patients and parents with pre-school children; evening and school holiday appointments for working patients and school children.

2. Patients who feel well may be unconvinced of the need to attend the clinic, so emphasise the importance of reviews even when feeling well. Linking clinic appointments to the time for repeat prescription revision is useful. Patients are likely to accept that they need to be seen for this purpose at least!

3. Adolescents and young adults may be reluctant attenders for scheduled doctors' appointments. A study by Price (1997) issued an invitation to 13, 15, and 17 year olds to visit their general practice for a health check. Three practices were involved: an inner city practice, a country town practice and a practice in a rural area. Seventy percent of the 13, 15 and 17 year olds attended this health check at which they talked about several health issues, including smoking. The study revealed that adolescents were more willing to talk about healthy living rather than disease. Ad hoc and opportunistic review may be the most effective ways of seeing these patients, who may attend the practice for other reasons eg for contraceptive advice. It is important to highlight in the notes or on the computer, that the patient needs an asthma review so that any member of the health care team can undertake this should they have an opportunity to do so.

4. It is always worth following non-attenders up with either a letter or a phone call. New approaches to these patients may be offered in the future with the use of the Internet and video phoning.

TRAINING (DOCTORS, NURSES AND SUPPORT STAFF)

Doctor training

Training in asthma care is available from a number of centres across the UK. The National Asthma and Respiratory Training Centre is the largest provider within the UK. Accredited and assessed distance learning programmes are available for doctors and nurses, these are often run in conjunction with local health authorities. Master degree courses and postgraduate diplomas are increasingly available for general practitioners. The GPs in Asthma Group (GPIAG) is a national special interest group of several hundred GPs. The group holds an annual educational conference and has a peer-review journal

Nurse training

If nurse training is required by the practice in order to provide preventive asthma care then funding and study time will need to be provided. Mentorship by the general practitioner, for the nurse who is undertaking training, is valuable and forms the framework for future referral procedures and expectations for the level of care that can be provided by the nurse working with autonomy. Nurses involved in running asthma clinics, or providing organised asthma care, must receive appropriate training and support. The National Asthma Task Force survey (Barnes & Partridge, 1993) revealed that 22% of asthma clinics were being run by untrained nurses.

The following guidelines on involvement of nurses in provision of care are provided by the National Asthma and Respiratory Training Centre.

Minimum involvement

At this level the practice nurse will undertake the following activities:

- compile an asthma register
- take a structured formal history
- take peak flow measurements in the surgery
- teach how to use a peak flow meter at home and how to chart a diary card
- demonstrate, instruct and check inhaler technique

The nurse should sit in with the GP or another asthma nurse specialist and observe consultations and should be encouraged to attend basic study days on asthma care.

Medium involvement

At this level the nurse undertakes all the minimum level activities plus the following:

- carry out diagnostic procedures (eg reversibility, exercise and serial peak flow monitoring)
- improve asthma education
- provide explanatory literature
- identify poor control, with referral back to the GP
- establish regular follow-up procedure

Again, sitting in on GP or asthma nurse consultations is beneficial. The nurse should undertake formal assessed training before developing their role further. Once this has been completed successfully, and further experience gained, the nurse is in a position to move on to a more autonomous role.

Maximum involvement

At this level the practice nurse should undertake all of the activities at minimum and medium level plus the following:

- carry out full assessment and regular follow-up
- formulate structured treatment plans in conjunction with the GP and patient
- prepare prescription for the GP to sign
- give telephone advice/additional appointments where appropriate
- see patients first in an emergency

Other personnel

It is helpful if other personnel receive basic training in the support of an asthma service. A receptionist should be aware of the particular needs of asthma patients, this includes:

- the need for asthma patients to receive an appointment within one week of discharge from the hospital or A&E
- if a patient has been seen during the night for their asthma, to receive an appointment for review the next day
- if an asthma patient has run out of inhalers, the

receptionist should get a prescription signed as soon as possible and the patient should be advised to make an appointment and/or ensure that they order their prescriptions in advance

- if a clinic appointment is cancelled the patient should be encouraged to book another one straight away
- if a patient phones for a repeat prescription for their inhaler, the receptionist should check which one they require to ensure that unnecessary scripts are not issued
- if a patient telephones and is breathless, and having difficulty speaking, the receptionist should put the call through to a doctor or an asthma nurse immediately

- persistent non-attenders at the asthma clinic or for a GP appointment should have their repeat prescription flagged with a note to say that they need to be seen before another prescription is issued

CONCLUSION

This chapter has described how the organisation of asthma care requires a commitment of time and personnel within the practice. It is an ongoing process which, if carried out effectively, can be immensely rewarding for the health professional in terms of improved patient outcomes and satisfaction.

10

RESEARCH AND AUDIT

INTRODUCTION – WHY?

Asthma is a researcher's dream. The cause of asthma is unknown, it affects over 5% of the population and it has no cure. Asthma offers endless possibilities to those whose penchant is audit: the disease affects all ages, has a variety of outcome measures, and costs the Health Service a great deal of money. Clearly one cannot function as a GP or practice nurse without at least some mild curiosity to learn more (research) or improve care (audit). This chapter is for health professionals who want to develop a research or audit interest, but wish for some gentle guidance. 'The yeti hypothesis' and 'Help yourself to an idea' sections are for enthusiasts.

The story of general practice research and audit in asthma, serves as an inspiration to doctors and nurses who believe good clinical research has its roots in the consulting room and not the ivory tower. Gregg's work in documenting peak flow rates is still the benchmark for respiratory clinics (Gregg, 1973). His epidemiological reviews are widely referenced 20 years on. Levy's work on diagnosis in children was accomplished, in a busy urban practice, without funding or external support (Levy and Bell, 1984). The classic education studies of Hilton and colleagues (Hilton et al., 1986) and Jenkinson and colleagues (Jenkinson et al., 1988) were UK general practice-based yet are internationally quoted as being definitive works on educational methods. Charlton's self-management plan (SMP) study (Charlton et al., 1990) was conducted within a single practice yet yielded more useful results than other larger academic studies (Hoskins et al., 1996). The whole nurse training movement began as a practice nurse's (Greta Barnes) 'good idea' and desire to help her colleagues (Barnes, 1985; Pearson, 1988). The Tayside Asthma Stamp had its origins in a practice where the GP and nurse (Anne Davidson and Jill Logan) held a joint clinic and needed to find a joint assessment tool (Neville, 1995).

The lesson from the past two decades of primary care research is simple: individual GPs and nurses can reshape the way we think and manage asthma. Try it.

GETTING STARTED

First of all you need a good idea. Ideas crop up during consultations, in the bath, on car journeys, whilst reading journals or, most commonly, chatting to colleagues. The evolution from idea to research, or audit proposal, can be laborious. Write down ideas. Let them lie for a day or two and see if they are worth pursuing. Try explaining your idea to a lay person, sceptical teenagers are ideal. Once you can describe your idea clearly and explain why it is important and how it could be done, you have the beginnings of a proposal.

The next step is to talk through your proposal with a fellow professional. A partner or close colleague will help you see potential pitfalls or tell you bluntly if your suggestion is a waste of time. After a few weeks of letting your idea/proposal mature it is time for some writing. Write down:

- a title
- what the proposal is about (introduction)
- how you want to do it (method)
- what you think you might find (results)
- how you will report this (analysis)
- what it might mean (discussion)

From now on you need a mentor. This can be a trainer, tutor, or local academic GP (see Table 10.1 – a vocabulary guide to help you talk to academics). A good mentor will let you make your own minor mistakes but stop you making major errors. A poor mentor will kill off your enthusiasm or try to take over your project.

There are short cuts to getting started from scratch. One simple method is to compare your practice asthma register with that of a neighbouring practice or with published work (Gellert et al., 1990). Perhaps your practice prevalence of asthma is lower than expected. Does this mean you are under-diagnosing cases? Could you have developed a useful system for taking 'asthmatics in remission' off your register? What does 'asthma in remission' mean - how many cases will become 'extinct' and how many 'erupt' in the future? Another starting point is to compare your prescribing trends with local or national trends (Naish et al., 1995; Griffiths et al., 1997). Do you use a wider range of inhaler devices than average? What percentage of your prescriptions are for preventive therapy? A computer search of patients who have been prescribed more than 12 bronchodilators inhalers in the past year is a useful place to begin an audit.

LITERATURE SEARCH

Split this task in two. The first phase is to look up review articles and key journal papers of direct relevance to your central theme. For example on 'education', look up Jenkinson's elegant study of video and audio tapes (Jenkinson et al., 1988). For 'diagnosis', check a medical textbook and read Speight's influential papers (Speight, 1978; Speight et al., 1983). It is easy to overdo a literature review and become disheartened because someone always seems to have done what you

Jargon	Meaning
p<0.05	1 in 20 chance of fluke result
p<0.01	1 in 100 chance of fluke result
p<0.001	1 in 1000 chance of fluke result, hence likely to be a true finding
Randomisation	Allocate to groups purely by chance (random is absolute, not relative)
Stratification	Group subjects by a characteristic (eg age) before randomising
Cohort	A group of people with a common feature followed over time
Odds Ratio (OR)	Comparison of observed with expected eg OR 1.0 = no difference, OR = 3 = large difference
95% Confidence Interval	There is 95% likelihood that the true result lies within these limits
Power calculation	The way of planning how many patients to include in a study
Internal validity	Results can be applied to the setting where the study was carried out eg practice
External validity	Results can apply to a wider population eg UK asthmatics
Prevalence	Number of cases in the population
Period prevalence	Number of cases present over a specified time eg one year
Incidence	New cases arising (usually per year) from a defined population
Meta analysis	Combined results of a number of studies involving one area of research eg bronchodilator treatments for asthma
Cross sectional analysis	Results compared with others produced at the same time
Longitudinal analysis	Comparison over time
SAMM Study	Safety Analysis of Marketed Medicines – the new term to replace Post Marketing Surveillance

Table 10.1 Jargon buster - a vocabulary guide to help you talk to academics

plan to do. In reality no one will have studied your problem in your practice. Ultimately, your interest lies in your practice and its population. Other peoples' findings will guide you but should not stop you exploring a problem for yourself.

The second phase of a literature review is a thorough search once your work is clearly defined. Try to find ten papers of direct relevance to your research or audit question. Define three 'key words' relevant to your topic eg asthma, diagnosis, general practice. Medline is available on private subscription or via medical libraries. If you are English speaking, restrict your search to the English language and the past 10 to 15 years only, unless you are exploring an unusual problem. Medline will give you abstracts of papers with the key words you specify. Obtain the full references from your library because the methodology section will be crucial in helping you see how others tackled your problem. The RCGP library offers members an excellent search facility supported by staff who are particularly experienced searching for medical papers (this is also available to non-members at an increased fee). The GPIAG Internet question answer service, lets you pose a question which an expert panel will answer, with key references if relevant (http://www.dundee.ac.uk/GeneralPractice/Asthma/welcome.htm). The Internet is gradually superseding other information systems; a search for key words eg asthma and research, will direct you to the world's top 20 asthma research units and literature services. Beware though - it is not subject to any validity controls.

Once you have read a reference keep a record on a card index or computer file. Use the Vancouver style, see the *BMJ* or the *British Journal of General Practice* (International Committee of Medical Journal Editors, 1988), note down the main points and anything which links you to the work eg you may know one of the authors or have trained at the hospital mentioned etc. Finally, the index of this book is a quick guide to key asthma references. The 'best' research papers of the past 20 years are listed in Ian Charlton's *Asthma in General Practice* review (Charlton, 1997) also available on the Internet http://www.gpiag-asthma.org/asthma/gpiag/jourindx.htm.

TYPES OF RESEARCH

Data collection

The simplest and easiest way to try out research or audit is to help a colleague. GPs are inundated with invitations to refer patients or collect cases for other people's research. One can learn a great deal from simply helping others, but insist on a few rules: ask to see the full protocol, ask for personalised feedback or results on your patients and ask for a copy of the final report or paper. Take your time with data work – inaccuracies can lead to misleading results. Inventing results is a very serious offence, of which the General Medical Council takes an equally serious view. The BMA recommend a fee of £9.50 for each patient form completed. Charge the full 'Insurance Medical Fee' for consultations specifically for a study. Make sure your collaborator has obtained Ethical Committee approval and make sure you have written informed consent from every patient involved in research. Audit, perceived as the practice of routine 'good care', does not generally require informed consent unless it concerns patients in additional activities to usual care.

Quantitative research

Quantitative studies concentrate on the collection and analysis of numerical data. A typical quantitative study will specify the number of participants from a defined population, will present data on the number of events occurring or some biological variable, and will include a statistical section containing p values or Odds Ratios. Analysis of morbidity trends, hospital admission rates, prescribing trends, peak flow or symptom scores are examples of quantitative research.

Qualitative research

In clinical work GPs and nurses can learn more from one patient studied in depth, than from several patients seen briefly. In research an interview with one or two patients can give insights into asthma care which yield more than reams of numeric data. Study of compliance, asthma and lifestyle, and health service utilisation are suited to a qualitative approach. Methods can include in-depth interviews, focus groups, participant observation and case studies. Good qualitative research is every bit as rigorous as good quantitative research and should not be viewed as an easier or more short-term route to answers. Very often, qualitative research leads to the generation of hypotheses that are then tested quantitatively.

Research networks

The Medical Research Council (MRC) and RCGP (Crombie and Fleming, 1986) run networks of practices to collaborate on issues such as hypertension management or 'Pill' safety. The routine chore of data collection is made worthwhile by research training for GPs and nurses, and invitations to seminars to discuss results. The GPIAG research network has produced influential work (Hoskins et al., 1996; Neville et al., 1993; Neville et al., 1997). It has a policy of providing practice and patient specific feedback to participants and results are presented at the GPIAG Annual Scientific Meetings.

Practices, with similar software, can collaborate in networks where study of prescribing is usually the focus. The Doctors Independent Network, GPASS in Scotland and the East London group are good examples. Here all data is automatically extracted without the need for form filling. NHS Research and Development (R&D) networks will gain in influence during the next decade, following Government commitment to support development of these in each health region. Practices that embark on research (not audit) associated with the award of peer-review grants are entitled to R&D funds through the 'Culyer' mechanisms to support their work. Ask your local R&D secretary (or nearest medical school) for details.

Cohort Studies

Cohort is a Roman military term now used to denote a group of subjects, with a shared characteristic, who are studied over time. Long-term cohort studies within a practice are immensely satisfying and strike a chord with GPs who care for their patients in a pastoral sense over a professional lifetime. Julian Tudor Hart (Tudor Hart, 1970) and John Fry (Fry, 1966) became internationally respected giants in their fields, not because they rattled off papers on esoteric subjects, but because they stayed put and used their lifelong commitment to their patients to produce first-rate studies. Many of the great unexplained problems of asthma research could be solved if more dedicated GPs observed their own patients' asthma relapses and remissions over their professional lifetimes (Spelman, 1984; Barritt and Davies, 1986; Price, 1995). Any takers?

Randomised controlled trial (RCT)

The RCT is regarded as the best way (gold standard) to assess whether a therapeutic intervention is effective. There are very strict rules on how RCTs should be conducted. Unless you know a statistician, have a substantial research grant, understand research ethics rules and have research experience, do not attempt an RCT! Within a research network they can be fascinating and rewarding but they are definitely not a solo pursuit. RCTs in primary care are of two types (Pringle and Churchill, 1995):

1. Within practice randomisation

Patients from the same practice are allocated to the intervention and the control groups. This works well for 'double blind' therapeutic trials but has problems of control contamination for 'non blind' interventions such as educational or behavioural studies (Hilton et al., 1986; White et al., 1989; Bryce et al., 1995; Levy et al., 1996; Feder et al., 1995).

2. Randomisation of entire practices

This can be problematic because there may be little incentive for a practice to enrol and then be classified as 'control'. Nevertheless, such studies are important when practice factors may be very influential in whether or not certain interventions are effective. A way round this problem is to have a phased intervention programme where 'control practices' test the intervention package after a time delay ('waiting list controls').

Questionnaires

Every year response rates from professionals and patients decline. Most questionnaires belong in the waste bin. The few that do not, are short (less than one page), easy to read (literacy level aged <8), clearly focused and have been refined after a pilot study.

Asthma researchers have a problem with assessing 'quality of life' for protocols. Hyland's (Hyland et al., 1991) 'asthma bother' questionnaire and St George's Respiratory Questionnaire are easy to use and validated. Questionnaire design is very difficult to do well and best left alone or to experts. Interviews within a practice yield much better data for research or audit purposes.

Analysis

We are used to complex analysis of large amounts of numeric data every time we inspect an ECG or peak flow chart. The 'eyeball technique' (a good long look) is an effective way to see if results are valid. Percentage predicted, peak flow bands are every day examples of applied statistics.

Analysis is all about whether results are internally valid and say something about the population they come from eg your practice, or externally valid and say something applicable to a wider audience. A review of peak flow charts on 20 of your patients will tell you (by 'eyeball') how many patients are stable and how many are at risk of attacks (percentage predicted). This would be an internally valid finding (you can apply it to your practice). External validity requires use of formal statistics. Refer to Swinscow's book for beginners (Swinscow, 1983) or Altman (Altman, 1991) for enthusiasts.

The joy of audit

Audit is an essential part of modern clinical practice but it can also be enjoyable if done with others and repeated! There are at least five reasons why asthma is a popular topic for audit:

1. It is common, presents at all ages, and at all times of the day and night. GP registrars must complete an audit project, and these features make asthma a popular choice of topic.
2. Nurse Asthma Diplomas also require an audit exercise.
3. Medical students like to study asthma.
4. Medical audit advisory groups encourage it.
5. Chronic Disease Management payment depends on it.

The real joy of audit is the comparison of results with other works or with your own work over time, 'cross sectional' and 'longitudinal' are the jargon terms (Barritt and Davies, 1986; Martys, 1992; Usherwood and Barber, 1988). 'Off the peg' audit packages save you the hassle of starting from scratch and give you an opportunity to compare your work with others. The East London practice network (Naish et al., 1995), Canterbury and Thanet audit (Pinnock, 1996) and GRASSIC (Grampian) (GRASSIC, 1994a; GRASSIC, 1994b) are good local packages. Bronchodilator/prescribing ratios can form a useful focus for audit. The Jones morbidity index (Jones et al., 1993) is popular. The pharmaceutical industry has a variety of packages of which the Action Asthma audit is best known. It is based on the Tayside Asthma Stamp. The GPIAG Research Unit has asthma attack and clinic management packages linked to patient specific feedback and comparison with national data. Computer enthusiasts can pit their wits against audit programmes developed in Southampton, Birmingham and Dundee (McCowan et al., 1997).

An intriguing finding from recent work is that practices with experience of audit, appear to have better patient outcomes (Neville et al., 1996). Audit enthusiasts will claim participation in audit improves care. Audit sceptics claim practices in the midst of improving care will enrol in audit as a means of effecting change. Does it matter whether good care is the result of audit or merely associated with it? Perhaps ask your patients.

Unfortunately, the NHS 1993 Chronic Disease Management accreditation system was based on measures of process (number of asthmatics in a practice, proportion on prophylactic therapy, percentage with peak flow recording) and not clinical outcome. Comparisons within and between practices are therefore flawed if based solely on these criteria. Audit work should look at structure, process and outcome (Usherwood and Barber, 1988; Pinnock, 1996). Measures of structure (relevant to general practice asthma care) are practice resources such as nebulisers and peak flow meters and measures of process refer to consultations and prescriptions.

OUTCOME MEASURES

There is as much disagreement on the definition of asthma as there is on what contributes to ideal outcome measures. All research and audit projects depend on a definition of outcome but unfortunately there are no universally accepted criteria. It is useful to establish markers of asthma care, and express outcome in terms of change in their use:

1. Hospital admission

Technically, one admission is a process but a reduction in numbers of admissions is desirable and 'an outcome'. A fall in re-admissions is generally accepted as a 'good outcome'.

2. Asthma attacks

GPIAG defines (Speight, 1978) these as '*an episode of respiratory symptoms which leads to an urgent consultations, increase or imitation of anti asthma therapy, and is associated with disruption to patient lifestyle eg loss of work, school or play*'. A reduction in the number of asthma attacks is a desirable outcome.

3. Bronchodilator/prophylactic ratio

Because this is easy to study (by use of PACT, see p21) it is popular as a marker of 'good care'. Practices with high levels of social deprivation have so called 'poor' bronchodilator/prophylactic ratios. Is this a marker of 'good patients' or 'good practices'?

4. Symptom scores

A fall in the number of patients within a practice who report having night-time, early morning or exercise cough wheeze, or breathlessness, is desirable and a reasonable marker of outcome.

5. Days lost

The number of days in the preceding month, when a patient has been unable to work/attend school/play, due to asthma, is a good marker of the impact of asthma on lifestyle. It is an easy to use outcome measure within practices. The drawback of this (and also the Jones morbidity index) is that up to 40% of patients will not attend work or school.

NURSE INVOLVEMENT IN RESEARCH AND AUDIT

Nursing is an emerging academic discipline and practice nursing is a relatively new occupation. Despite this, nurses have made a major contribution to research and audit during the past 20 years. Nurses are generally better than doctors at working to protocols and assessing patients in a structured manner.

Nurses run most practice asthma audits. A difficulty many nurses face is trying to obtain a practice consensus on asthma management. Audit can be a useful objective way to show GPs within a practice how they manage problems. Nurses, working with an asthma interested partner, can use audit findings to help less enthusiastic partners to develop the skills needed to manage asthma attacks and routine care. A simple audit of antibiotic prescribing rates in asthmatic children, by a partner, is a good way to initiate debate. Nurse-run audit and presentation of results is also a subtle way of giving GPs the confidence to refer patients to the nurse for routine follow-up and management according to guidelines.

Research studies have shown that respiratory nurses can reduce post-admission morbidity. There have been no clinical trials on nurse versus no nurse management in a practice. The Bryce and colleagues facilitator study (Bryce et al., 1995) did show that those children invited to a nurse-run asthma clinic did better than controls after 12 months. Circumstantial evidence suggests that nurse-run clinics are associated with favourable outcome. Hoskins and colleagues have shown that patients, managed by practices with a nurse with a recognised asthma diploma, do better than those managed by other nurses (Hoskins et al.,1998). This may mean that practices with 'good asthma care' send their nurses on training programmes or that nurses with a diploma manage patients better, or both.

Practice nurses could contribute more to research if adequately trained and supported. Does nurse support and follow-up improve the care of patients with 'brittle asthma'? Is nurse care less expensive than GP care? Should nurses prescribe salbutamol, terbutaline, beclomethasone and budesonide within set dosage limits? Do patients tell their nurse the truth about compliance with medication?

FUNDING

Self funding (£0)

'Unfunded research' is a misnomer. Research without external support means work in leisure time and resources taken from NHS practice (telephone, stationery and typing). Before embarking on unsupported research it is worth setting a limit to your time and resource commitment. It may even be politic to negotiate this with your family. Some of the classic long-term follow-up studies from general practice are 'unfunded'. Funding can sometimes impose deadlines and the necessity to produce reports. Some amateur research enthusiasts choose to do unfunded research precisely because it is an interest to be pursued at one's own pace.

Research donations (<£1,000)

A one off donation can be very helpful to buy equipment (spirometer or nebulisers), organise travel to meetings or a presentation (to cover cost of slides or poster preparation). Local pharmaceutical industry representatives are an option here, but it is best to avoid taking any donations linked to work on prescribing. Sums of above £1,000 are best sought as grants rather than donations.

Modest grants (£1,000 - £10,000)

Projects that require a commitment of medical, nursing or auxiliary staff time, or purchases of computers, need external grant funding. Medical and nursing time can be calculated as locum equivalent time. This will keep partners happy if you reduce clinical commitments to pursue research. Sources of modest grants are the BMA, the RCGP and local R&D networks. Forms need to be filled, references found, polite letters written and end of project reports completed. Those issuing grants quite rightly expect a research report and a presentation or paper based on your work. You will need friendly advice on how to word applications. Try to make your application accessible and readable to non-experts, particularly as most grant bodies contain lay members. Most small grant applications underestimate resources (remember holidays, stationary, telephone calls and travel). Grant bodies do not like paying for new computers. If you intend to employ staff think seriously about involving a university department of general practice and/or primary care.

Major grants (>£10,000)

Work involving the employment of new staff – nurses, data processors, secretaries – should be done through a university department. Research is difficult enough without dealing with employment law, salaries and insurance cover. Major grants take a long time to prepare. Keep the idea simple, stick to one hypothesis and follow the grant givers' rules and procedures to the letter. You will almost certainly need multidisciplinary collaboration and statistical help. It is even worth considering the likes and dislikes of grant giving bodies (see Table 10.2).

Costing studies requires care and as a rule, randomised controlled therapeutic trials need approximately £1,000 per patient and national collaborations need at least £50,000 annually. Major grants imply a commitment to produce annual reports, presentations at meetings and publications in peer-review journals. Always acknowledge your sponsor.

The 'big sponsors' of UK asthma research are the National Asthma Campaign (£3 million annually), Medical Research Council, NHS R&D, and the Chief Scientist's Office in Scotland. The larger pharmaceutical firms – Glaxo Wellcome, Astra, 3M, Zeneca, MSD, Boehringer – have a substantial commitment to supporting good primary care research, in addition to their own very large R&D programmes. Approach companies via their medical divisions and not their local sales representatives.

ETHICAL APPROVAL

Audit does not usually need Ethical Committee approval but research always does; if in doubt, apply. Every district is covered by a committee made up of academic and clinical experts with lay representatives. Unfortunately, committees all have different forms, rules and criteria. Some charge applicants, others do not. Speak with your local secretary before submitting a proposal otherwise you will waste their time and yours.

Likes	Dislikes
Multidisciplinary	Single author applications
Collaboration	Solo working
One hypothesis	Lots of aims
Statistical power calculations	Typing errors
Accurate references	Buying computers
Results of pilot work	Unknown GPs
Plan for disseminating findings	Arithmetic errors
Timetable	Extra pages included
A lay reader's summary	'Soft' outcomes
Famous 'experts' as applicants	Inexperienced applicants
Hard outcome measures	

Table 10.2 Likes and dislikes of research funding bodies

Applications need to include a full protocol and a lay summary (Smith et al., 1997). Consent forms are needed. Research involving children, or persons with a reduced decision making capacity, or in a dependent relationship to the researcher, need special consideration. Grant awards are never made without formal approval. Make sure you have seen the ethics approval if you participate in a collaborative project.

When preparing an ethics application it is helpful to ask yourself two simple questions:

- could I defend what I propose to do on live TV?
- would I be happy for my patients to know what I am doing?

Medical defence unions will offer cover for research that has received Ethical Committee approval.

SPREAD THE WORD

Research and audit will increase your knowledge and expertise. You have a professional obligation to share your findings with as wide an audience as you can. The people you work with and the persons you studied have a right to see your findings. Grant awards are accompanied by a commitment to present and to publish. However, be very cautious about talking to the media before you are in print, as there are strict rules on pre-publication release of results, and you may find your prestigious paper rejected on these grounds.

Presentation

In-practice asthma audits are ideal for weekly or monthly practice team meetings. You can stimulate debate by circulating a results summary. It is useful, not to say polite, to present your work to your friends and immediate colleagues first. They may tolerate your hesitancies and may offer friendly criticism. The box below includes some of the best national fora for prescribing work on asthma.

RCGP Meetings	Formal and constructive criticism
AUDGP Conference	Peer-reviewed, tough academic criticism
GPIAG	Peer-reviewed but friendly and fun (the organisers will even make your slides!)
BTS	Large, intimidating and sometimes harsh
NAC	Large, intimidating but polite and friendly

BMJ	The highest impact, but with a very low acceptance rate!
British Journal of General Practice	High standard required and fierce competition (they receive lots of asthma papers compared to other subjects).
Thorax, Respiratory Medicine, European Respiratory Journal	High impact factor but readership is mainly chest physicians.
Asthma in General Practice (GPIAG), Asthma Journal (NAC)	Ideal for primary care work whether single practice or larger studies
The Practitioner, Update, Prescriber	Supportive editors, wide GP readership but little impact on respiratory 'decision makers'
Pulse, Doctor, GP News	Suitable for case studies or opinion, not original research
Internet (GPIAG site)	A novel way to spread the word

Publication

Writing up projects is beyond the scope of this chapter. The box above includes the best publications to aim papers on asthma care.

OVERCOMING THE HURDLES

There will probably be occasions when you come up against problems or resistance to your study. Table 10.3 highlights some of the potential problems and suggests solutions.

THE YETI HYPOTHESIS

A yeti is a mysterious creature which wanders around the high Himalayas and is never seen. The yeti hypothesis states that some multifactorial diseases have a major unknown risk factor or cause. The peptic ulcer disease, 'yeti', was Helicobacter Pyloridi. Sleeping position was the mysterious 'yeti' contributing to sudden infant death syndrome.

Problem	Suggestion
Partners are not interested	Present comparative data to demonstrate the problem
No funding	Ask for a local donation
Journal rejection	Ask a colleague to criticise then submit elsewhere (even best selling authors receive rejections)
Poor recruitment	Stop the study and write up as a pilot
'Condition becomes rare'	We often decide to study problems at times of peak incidence then do the study when incidence is declining
Ethical Committee refusal	Have a complete re-think!

Table 10.3 Crisis resolution table

Is there an asthma 'yeti'? One cannot explain the incidence and prevalence of asthma on the known risk factors of genetic risk and allergens. Dietary factors may explain some of the recent rise in prevalence: is high sodium intake the asthma yeti? Many children have no genetic susceptibility to asthma yet have a cough, wheeze and breathlessness following upper respiratory infection. Is there an undiscovered 'yeti' virus? Does the late fetal environment pre-programme lung growth and the immune system to develop asthma?

Like the Himalayan yeti, medical yetis are fun to look for, rarely seen and almost never caught.

HELP YOURSELF TO AN IDEA

The best ideas for research and audit come from everyday clinical problems. The following list consists of unsolved puzzles which are likely to be tackled and answered within the next ten years (Barnes, 1993). Research committees and grant givers will be interested to receive bids to explore the following:

- when should patients 'step down' their anti-asthma therapy?
- do inhaled steroids alter the natural history of asthma?
- is there a blood or sputum biochemical marker of asthma inflammation?
- which asthma patients need follow-up and how often?
- which patients will benefit from leukotriene antagonists?
- can inhaled steroids be used on an 'as required' basis in childhood upper respiratory infections?
- can the outcome of 'brittle asthma' be modified by a behavioural approach?
- will patients use an Internet-based virtual asthma clinic?

APPENDIX 1

ASTHMA CLINIC PROTOCOL: AN EXAMPLE FRAMEWORK

(Modified with advice from Greta Barnes SRN MBE)

1. Objectives
a) To gain rapid control of symptoms
b) To maximise lifestyle by abolishing symptoms through minimum treatment
c) To reduce acute asthma attacks, and therefore hospital admission
d) To facilitate self-management by patients
e) To encourage patient education

2. Equipment, drugs and systems
Suitable room
Steriliser (for mouthpieces)
Height measure (*Stadiometer)
Weighing scales
Appointment system
Asthma and COPD Register
Record cards (eg those supplied by the National Asthma and respiratory Training Centre (NARTC), Warwick
Telephone

Peak flow meters and stethoscopes
Spirometer (In order to diagnose COPD)
Written learning materials and leaflets
Peak flow charts
Self-management plans
Placebo inhaler devices

Oxygen
High flow oxygen regulator* (to drive nebulisers)
Beta-2 agonist bronchodilators (pMDI inhalers and nebuliser solution)
Oral steroid tablets
Nebuliser(s)
Compressor(s)

3. Selection of patients
a) From prescription requests
b) By referral from general practitioner

(* = optional desirable items)

c) Through follow-up from out of hours intervention
d) By referral following opportunistic detection
d) By self-referral.

4. Diagnosis
a) History and symptoms
b) Peak flow monitoring (15% variation)
c) Reversibility testing
d) Exercise test
e) Therapy trial (inhaled or oral steroid trial)

Early detection through case finding or screening
a) Opportunistic
b) Notes search
c) New registrations
d) Health promotion

5. Management
First visit
History
    Provocation (trigger factors)
    Present symptoms
    Other medical conditions and drug therapy
    Height
    Weight (percentile chart for children)
Confirm diagnosis (see Chapter 4):
    Peak expiratory flow reversibility test
    Diary cards
Identify, demonstrate and teach appropriate delivery system (see Chapter 8)
Prescribe medication at step appropriate to severity (see Chapters 5 and 7)
Give treatment card/peak flow meter cards as appropriate
Follow-up appointment initially after two weeks
Education and provide basic self-management plan (see Chapter 7)

Follow-up
Timing
a) Seasonal/very mild = 1 year
b) Mild to moderate = 3-6 months
c) Severe = 1-3 months.

At each visit

a) Monitor symptoms, usage of beta-2 agonist bronchodilators, exercise tolerance and quality of life
b) Check days off work/school due to asthma
c) Take peak flow and check peak flow record
d) Take lowest and highest peak flow reading for last two weeks to calculate percentage variation
e) Check inhaler technique and compliance
f) Check growth (in children use percentile chart)
g) Adjust treatment as necessary
h) Try to elicit information on the patients understanding of asthma and reinforce appropriately

6. Education

Try to establish what the patient wants to know and tailor the education accordingly.

Every patient should be aware of the following points on leaving the clinic:

a) How to tell when their asthma is going out of control:
1. by monitoring peak flow
2. increase in symptoms
3. decrease in effectiveness of medication

b) When to call for help
c) How the asthma drugs work
d) How to monitor peak flow for moderate and severe asthmatics, including all patients who have had an acute severe attack, have been nebulised or have been given oral steroids. Mild asthmatics who are highly motivated may also wish to do this
e) How to exercise their respiratory muscles
f) About smoking (don't)
g) About the National Asthma Campaign

7. Treatment pathway

Tailor treatment according to published guidelines (The British Thoracic Society 1997, Spelman 1996, Scheffer 1995, 2281, 102, 24).

8. Referral

(and consultation with general practitioner when in doubt)

Initially, clinics should be run jointly by the nurse and the doctor. Criteria for referrals are as follows:

Referrals from the practice nurse to the general practitioner

a) Peak flow reduced by 50%
b) Excessive use of reliever drugs
c) Difficult to control despite adequate treatment
d) An incomplete response to treatment
e) Evidence or suspicion of concurrent illness
f) At patient request
g) Emergency attendances
h) Any patients on beta-blockers/NSAIDS
i) Suspected occupational asthma

Referrals to practice nurse

a) Self
b) From general practitioner
   1. new patients
   2. for education/assessment of inhaler technique
c) Nurse to nurse
d) Receptionist
e) In absence of doctor in emergency

Referrals to hospital (see Chapter 6)

a) Patients not responding to emergency therapy (peak flow up by 15% at least) or with PEF below 50% best or predicted
b) Patients requiring daily or regular oral steroids
c) Failure to respond to adequate (non-emergency) treatment
d) Children on high doses of inhaled steroids
e) Where there are difficulties with diagnosis

Referrals to others

a) National Asthma Campaign
b) Anti-smoking groups
c) Dietitian/obesity clinic
d) Occupational physician.

9. Audit

Subjects suitable for audit include:

a) Acute asthma attacks
b) Use of nebulisers (emergency and regular)
c) Use of short course of steroids
d) Home visits
e) Hospital admissions and re-admissions
f) Incidence and prevalence of asthma in practice
g) Percentage of patients on prophylaxis
h) Clinic/surgery non-attenders

APPENDIX 2

FURTHER INFORMATION

Useful addresses

British Allergy Foundation
Deepdene House
30 Bellegrove Road
Welling
Kent DA16 3PY

Telephone: 0181 303 8525
Fax: 0181 303 8792
Email: allergybaf@compuserve. com
Website: www.allergyfoundation.com

British Lung Foundation
78 Hatton Garden
London EC1N 8LD

Telephone: 0171 831 5831
Fax: 0171 831 5832
Website: www.lunguk.org/
welcome.htm

British Thoracic Society
6th Floor, North Wing
New Garden House
78 Hatton Garden
London EC1M 8JR

Telephone: 0171 831 8788
Fax: 0171 831 8766

Chest Heart and Stroke Association
65 North Castle Street
Edinburgh
EH2 3LT

Telephone: 0131 225 6963
Fax: 0131 220 6313
Email: chss@dial.pipex.com

Cochrane Airways Group
Department of Public Health
Sciences
St George's Hospital Medical
School
Cranmer Terrace
London SW17 0RE

Telephone: 0181 725 2790
Fax: 0181 725 3584
Email: airways@sghms.ac.uk

General Practitioners in Asthma
Group (GPIAG)
MMI
Bath Brewery
Toll Bridge Road
Bath BA1 7DE

Website: www.gpiag-asthma.org/
asthma/GPIAG/welcome.htm

GPIAG Research Unit
Tayside Centre for General Practice
Kirsty Semple Way
Dundee DD2 4AD

Telephone: 01382 632805
Fax: 01382 633839
Website: www.dundee.ac.uk/
GeneralPractice/Asthma/
welcome.htm

Health Education Authority
Trebelyan House
30 Great Peter St
London SW1P 2HW

Telephone: 0171 222 5300
Fax: 0171 413 8900
Website: www.hea.org.uk

National Asthma Campaign
Providence House
Providence Place
London N1 0NT

Telephone: 0171 226 2260
Fax: 0171 704 0740
Website: www.asthma.org.uk

- Educational material for health
professional and patients with
asthma as well as their families,
speakers for meetings, advice

- Telephone help line or 0845 701
0203
- Social and fundraising meetings
- Research
- The Junior Asthma Club

For information on the NAC
Professional Subscription Scheme:
National Asthma Campaign
FREEPOST ANG 2568
Finchingfield
Braintree CM7 4BR

National Asthma & Respiratory
Training Centre
The Athenaeum
10 Church Street
Warwick CV34 4AB

Telephone: 01926 493313
Fax: 01926 493224
Email: enquiries@nartc.org.uk

- Courses for nurses and doctors
on asthma
- Correspondence course
including Diploma recognised
by the Royal College of General
Practitioners
- Asthma clinic record cards for sale
- Masters level, distance learning
Diploma in Primary Care
Respiratory Medicine (jointly with
St George's Hospital Medical
School, University of London)

Commercial companies

3M Health Care
Morley Street
Loughborough
Leics LE11 1EP

Telephone: 01509 611611
Fax: 01509 237288
Website: www.3m.com/uk

- Asthma drugs
- Aerochamber spacer device

Astra Pharmaceuticals Ltd
Home Park Estate
Kings Langley
Herts WD4 8DH

Telephone: 01923 266191
Fax: 01923 260431
Website: www.astra.com

- Educational material
- Nurse training courses
- Clinic materials
- McCarthy masks for Nebuhalers
- Stickers for children
- Triflo inhalation teaching aid
- Peak flow whistles

Baker Norton Ltd
Albert Basin
Royal Docks
London E16 2QJ

Telephone: 08705 020304
Fax: 08705 323334

BASICS
7 Black Hurse Lane
Ipswich IP1 2EF

Telephone: 01473 218407
Fax: 01473 280585
Website: www.basics.freeserve.com

BOC Gases
The Priestley Centre
10 Priestley Road
Surrey Research Park
Guildford
Surrey GU2 5XY

Telephone: 0800 111333
Fax: 0800 111555
Email: customer.service@uk.gases.
   boc.com

- Oxygen supplies

Boehringer Ingelheim Ltd
Ellesfield Avenue
Bracknell
Berkshire RG12 8YS

Telephone: 01344 424600
Fax: 01344 741444

Website: www.boehringer-ingelheim.
   com

Clement Clarke
Edinburgh Way
Harlow
Essex CM20 2TT

Telephone: 01279 414969
Fax: 01279 635232
Website: www.clement-clarke.com

- Peak flow meters
- Spirometers
- In-check device
- Flutter device

Ferraris Medical Ltd
Ferraris House
Aden Road
Enfield
Middlesex EN3 7SE

Telephone: 0181 805 9055
Fax: 0181 805 9065
Email: ferraris@globalnet.co.uk

- Peak flow meters

Glaxo Wellcome UK Ltd
Stockley Park West
Uxbridge
Middlesex UB11 1BT

Telephone: 0181 990 9888
Fax: 0181 990 4321
Website: www.glaxowellcome.co.uk

- Practice nurse courses
  (respiratory care team)
- Educational material for health
  professionals and patients
  (Action Asthma)
- Clinic start-up packs
- (Tayside record stamp – Action
  Asthma)

Jaeger (UK)
Millers House
Roman Way
Market Harborough
Leicestershire LE16 7PQ

Telephone: 01858 433344

Fax: 01858 410185
Email: jjs@jaeger-
   uk.ccmail.compuserve.com

- Spirometers

Medic-Aid Ltd
Heath Place
Bognor Regis
W Sussex
PO22 9SL

Telephone: 01243 846111 or
   01243 840888
Fax: 01243 846100
Email: customer.service@medic-aid.
   com
Website: www.medic-aid.com

- Nebulisers

Merck Sharpe & Dohme
Hertford Road
Hoddesdon
Hertfordshire EN11 9BU

Telephone: 01992 467272
Fax: 01992 451066
Website: www.merck.com

- Leucotriene receptor
- Antagonist drugs

Micro-Medical
6 Ambley Green
Gillingham Business Park
Gillingham
Kent ME8 0NJ

Telephone: 01634 360044
Fax: 01634 36005
Email: sales@micromed.co.uk
Website: www.micromed.co.uk

- Peak flow meters/spirometers

ML Laboratories
60 London Lane
St Albans
Hertfordshire AL1 1NG

Telephone: 01727 837341
Fax: 01727 837345

- Clickhaler

Napp Pharmaceuticals
Cambridge Science Park
Milton Road
Cambridge
CB4 0GW
Telephone: 01223 424444
Fax: 01223 424441

Ohmeda
Ohmeda House
71 Great North Road
Hatfield
Herts
AL9 5EN

Telephone: 01707 263570
Fax: 01707 260065

- Oximeters

Rhone-Polenc Rorer
RPR House
50 Kings Hill Avenue
West Malling
Kent ME19 4AH

Telephone: 01732 584000
Fax: 01732 584080
Website: www.rp-rorer.com
- Educational material
- Spinhaler whistles and connectors for Nebuhalers
- Courses for nurses

Schering-Plough
Schering-Plough House
Shire Park
Welwyn Garden City
Herts AL7 1TW

Telephone: 01707 363636
Fax: 01509 237288
Website: schering-plough.com

- Allergy, asthma and rhinitis drugs

Zeneca Pharmaceuticals
Kings Court
Water Lane
Wilmslow
Cheshire SK9 5AZ

Telephone: 01625 712712
Fax: 01625 712532

- Leucotriene receptor
- Antagonist drugs

REFERENCES

Agertoft L and Pedersen S (1993). Importance of the inhalation device on the effect of budesonide. *Archives of Disease in Childhood* **69**(1): 130-133

Allen SC (1988). Missed asthma: a study in 13 old people. *British Journal of Clinical Practice* **42**(4): 158-160

Altman DG (1991). *Practical Statistics for Medical Research*. London, Chapman and Hall

Anderson HR (1989). Increase in hospital admissions for childhood asthma: trends in referral, severity and readmissions from 1970 to 1985 in a health region of the United Kingdom. *Thorax* **44**(8): 614-9

Anderson HR, Bland JM and Peckham CS (1987). Risk factors for asthma up to 16 years of age. Evidence from a national cohort study. *Chest* **91**(6 suppl): 127S-130S

Anderson HR, Butland BK and Strachan DP (1994a). Trends in the prevalence and severity of childhood asthma. *British Medical Journal* **308**: 1600-4

Anderson HR, Esmail A, Hollowell J et al., (1994b). Lower respiratory disease. In: Stevens A, Raftery J (Eds). *Health care needs assessment* **1**: 256-332. Radcliffe Medical Press, Oxford

Anderson HR, Pottier AC and Strachan DP (1992). Asthma from birth to age 23: incidence and relation to prior and concurrent atopic disease. *Thorax* **47**(7): 537-42

Anonymous (1990). Guidelines for the management of asthma in adults: II – Acute severe asthma. Statement by the British Thoracic Society, the Research Unit of the Royal College of Physicians of London, the King's Fund Centre and the National Asthma Campaign [published erratum in *British Medical Journal* 1990 **301**(6755): 797-800]

Anonymous (1993). Guidelines on the management of asthma. Statement by the British Thoracic Society, the British. Paediatric Association, the Research Unit of the Royal College of Physicians of London, the King's Fund Centre, the National Asthma Campaign, the Royal College of General Practitioners, the General Practitioners in Asthma Group, the British Association of Accident and Emergency Medicine, and the British Paediatric Respiratory Group [published errata appear in *Thorax* 1994 **49**(1): 96 and 1994 **49**(4): 386]. *Thorax* **48**(2 suppl): S1-24

Anonymous (1993). International consensus report on diagnosis and treatment of asthma. National Heart, Lung, and Blood Institute, National Institutes of Health. Bethesda, Maryland 20892. Publication no. 92 3091, March 1992. *European Respiratory Journal* **5**(5): 601-641

Auty RM and Holgate ST (1989). Nedocromil sodium: a review of its anti-inflammatory properties and clinical activity in the treatment of asthma. In: Kay AB (Ed) *Allergy and Asthma: New trends and approaches to therapy*, pp 171-188. London Academic Press

Barnes G (1985). Nurse-run asthma clinics in general practice. *Journal of the Royal College of General Practitioners* **35**(278): 447

Barnes G, Booker R and Brown (1997). Devices under discussion. pp1-8. Warwick, UK. National Asthma and Respiratory Training Centre

Barnes G and Partridge MR (1994). Community asthma clinics: 1993 survey of primary care by the National Asthma Task Force *Quality in Health Care* **3**: 133-136

Barnes PJ (1993). Asthma: what is there left to find out? *British Medical Journal* **307**: 814-815

Barritt P and Davies R (1986). Measuring success in asthma care. *Family Practice* **3**(4): 229-34

Beasley R, Burgess C, Pearce N et al., (1994). Confounding by severity does not explain the association between fenoterol and asthma death. *Clinical & Experimental Allergy* **24**(7): 660-668

Beasley R, Cushley M and Holgate ST (1989). A self management plan in the treatment of adult asthma. *Thorax* **44**: 200-204

Beer S, Laver J, Karpuch J et al., (1987). Prodromal features of asthma. *Archives of Disease in Childhood* **62**(4): 345-348

Bellamy D and Ed Levy M (1998). Nebuliser Factsheet. http://www.gpiag-asthma.org/asthma/GPIAG/welcome.htm: General Practitioners in Asthma Group

Bernard-Bonnin AC, Stachenko S, Bonin D et al., (1995). Self-management teaching programs and morbidity of pediatric asthma: a meta-analysis. *Journal of Allergy and Clinical Immunology* **95**(1 pt 1): 34-41

Bevis M and Taylor B (1990). What do school teachers know about asthma? *Archives of Disease in Childhood* **65**: 622-5

Blake KV, Hoppe M , Harman E et al., (1992). Relative amount of albuterol delivered to lung receptors from a metered dose inhaler and nebuliser solution. *Chest* **101**(2): 309-15

Borgstrom L and Newman S (1993) Total and regional lung deposition of terbutaline sulphate inhaled via a pressurised MDI or via Turbohaler. *International Journal of Pharmaceutics.* **97**(pt1/3): 47-53

Borgstrom L, Derom E, Stahl E et al., (1996) The inhalation device influences lung deposition and bronchodilating effect of terbutaline. *American Journal of Respiratory Critical Care Medicine* **153**(5): 1636-1640

British Thoracic Association (1982). Death from asthma in two regions. *British Medical Journal* **285**: 1251-1255

British Thoracic Society and others (1993). Guidelines for the management of asthma: a summary. *British Medical Journal* **306**: 776-782

Bryce FP, Neville RG, Crombie IK et al., (1995). Controlled trial of an audit facilitator in diagnosis and treatment of childhood asthma in general practice. *British Medical Journal* **310**: 838-842

Bucknall CE, Robertson C, Moran F et al., (1988a). Management of asthma in hospital: a prospective audit. *British Medical Journal* **296**: 1637-1639

Bucknall CE, Robertson C, Moran F et al., (1988b). Differences in hospital asthma management. *Lancet* **1**: 748-750

Burr ML, Butland BK, King S et al., (1989). Changes in asthma prevalence: two surveys 15 years apart. *Archives of Diseases in Childhood* **64**(10): 1452-6

Burr ML, Charles TJ, Roy K et al., (1979). Asthma in the elderly: an epidemiological survey. *British Medical Journal* **1**: 1041-1044

Cates CJ (1998). Comparison of holding chambers and nebulisers for beta-agonists in acute asthma (Cochrane Review). Issue 2: Update Software. Oxford, Update Software

Charlton I (1997). The contribution primary care (general practice) has made to asthma care in the past years. *Asthma in General Practice* **5**(2): 18-20

Charlton I, Charlton G, Broomfield J et al., (1991). Audit of the effect of a nurse run asthma clinic on workload and patient morbidity in general practice. *British Journal of General Practice* **41**(347): 227-31

Charlton I and Charlton G (1990). New perspectives in asthma self-management. *Practitioner* **234**: 30-32

Charlton I and Charlton G (1994). Caring for patients with asthma. Teaching self management takes time [letter; comment]. *British Medical Journal* **308**: 1370-1371

Charlton I, Antoniou AG, et al., (1994). Asthma at the interface: bridging the gap between general practice and a district general hospital. *Archives of Disease in Childhood* **70**(4): 313-318

Charlton I, Charlton G, Broomfield J et al., (1990). Evaluation of peak flow and symptoms only self-management plans for control of asthma in general practice. *British Medical Journal* **301**: 1355-9

Charlton I, Charlton G, Broomfield J et al., (1991). Audit of the effect of a nurse run asthma clinic on workload and patient morbidity in a general practice. *British Journal of General Practice* **41**: 227-31.

Charlton I, Jones K and Bain J (1991). Delay in diagnosis of childhood asthma and its influence on respiratory consultation rates. *Archives of Disease in Childhood* **66**(5): 633-635

Chung KF (1986). Role of imflammation in the hyperreactivity of the airways in asthma. Editorial. *Thorax* **41**: 657-62

Cockcroft DW, Killian DN, Mellon JJA et al., (1977). Bronchial reactivity to inhaled histmine; a method and clinical survey. *Clinical Allergy* **7**: 235-43

Collier J and Hilton SR (1998). Doctors and patients should sign prescriptions. *British Medical Journal* **317**: 951

Committee on the Safety of Medicines, Rawlins M (Chair) (1992). Report of the beta-agonist working party. London. Committee on Safety of Medicines

Crombie DL and Fleming DM (1986). The Third National Study of Morbidity Statistics from General Practice. *Journal of the Royal College of General Practitioners*. Editorial. **36**(283): 51-52

Crosby FRG, Whyte E, Ogston S et al., (1989). Improving asthma control in general practice. *Thorax* **44**: 344

David TJ, Wybrew M and Hennessen U (1984). Prodromal itching in childhood asthma. *Lancet* **21**(2): 154-155

Dickinson J, Hutton S, Atkin A et al., (1997). Reducing asthma morbidity in the community: the effect of a targeted nurse-run asthma clinic in an English general practice. *Respiratory Medicine* **91**(10): 634-640

Dickinson J, Hutton S and Atkin A (1998). Implementing the British Thoracic Society's guidelines: the effect of a nurse-run asthma clinic on prescribed treatment in an English general practice. *Respiratory Medicine* **92**: 264-267

Douglas JG, Rafferty P, Fergusson RJ et al., (1985). Nebulised salbutamol without oxygen in severe acute asthma: how effective and how safe? *Thorax* **40**(3): 180-183

Drever F, Bunting J and Harding D (1997). Male mortality from major causes of death. In: Drever F, Whitehead M (Eds). *Health inequalities*. The Stationery Office, London.

D'Souza W, Burgess C, Ayson M et al., (1996). Trial of a "credit card" asthma self-management plan in a high-risk group of patients with asthma. *Journal of Allergy & Clinical Immunology* **97**(5): 1085-1092

D'Souza W, Crane J, Burgess C et al.,(1994). Community-based asthma care: trial of a "credit card" asthma self-management plan. *European Respiratory Journal* **7**(7): 1260-1265

Djukanovic WR, Roche WR and Holgate ST (1989). Bronchial inflammation as an underlying mechanism of asthma and its clinical consequences. *Hospital Update* **15**: 266-81

Eason J and Markowe HJL (1987). Controlled investigation of deaths from asthma in hospitals in the North-East Thames region. *British Medical Journal* **294**: 1255-1258

Edwards AGK, Russell IT and Stott NCH (1998). Signal versus noise in the evidence base for medicine: an alternative to hierarchies of evidence. *Family Practice* **15**(4): 319-323

Ellis ME and Friend JAR (1985). How well do asthma clinic patients understand their asthma? *British Journal of Diseases of the Chest* **79**: 43-8

Ernst P, Fitzgerald JM and Spier S (1996). Canadian Asthma Consensus Conference: Summary of recommendations. *Canadian Respiratory Journal* **3**(2): 89-100

Evans D, Clark NM and Feldman CH (1987). School health education programmes for asthma. *Clinical Reviews in Allergy* **5**: 207-12

Feder G, Griffiths C, Highton C et al., (1995). Do clinical guidelines introduced with practice based education improve care of asthmatic and diabetic patients? A randomised controlled trial in general practices in east London. *British Medical Journal* **311**: 1473-8

Fireman P, Friday GA, Gira C et al., (1981). Teaching self-management skills to asthmatic children and their parents in an ambulatory care setting. *Pediatrics* **68**: 341-8

Fish JE, Kemp JP, Lockey RF et al., (1997). Zafirlukast for symptomatic mild-to-moderate asthma: A 13-week multicenter study. *Clinical Therapeutics* **19**(4): 675-690

Fletcher HJ, Ibrahim SA and Speight N (1990). Survey of asthma deaths in the Northern region, 1970-85. *Archives of Disease in Childhood* **65**(2): 163-167

Fry J (1966). *Profiles of Disease*. A study in the Natural History of Common Diseases. Edinburgh, Livingstone

Fuller RW (1996). The asthma death problem revisited. *British Journal of Clinical Pharmacology* **42**(1): 11-14

Garrett JE, Lanes SF, Kolbe J et al., (1996). Risk of severe life threatening asthma and beta agonist type: an example of confounding by severity. *Thorax* **51**(11): 1093-1099

Geelhoed GC, Landau LI and Le Souef PN (1994). Evaluation of SaO2 as a predictor of outcome in 280 children presenting with acute asthma. *Annals of Emergency Medicine* **23**(6): 1236-1241

Gellert AR, Gellert SL and Iliffe SR (1990). Prevalence and management of asthma in a London inner city general practice. *British Journal of General Practitioners* **40**: 197-201

Gibson GJ (1996). *Clinical tests of respiratory function.* 2nd edn. London, Chapman and Hall Medical

Gleeson JG, Green S and Price JF (1988). Air or oxygen as driving gas for nebulised salbutamol. *Archives of Disease in Childhood* **63**(8): 900-904

Grampian Asthma Study of Integrated Care (GRASSIC) (1994). Effectiveness of routine self-monitoring of peak flow in patients with asthma. *British Medical Journal* **308**: 564-567

Grampian Asthma Study of Integrated Care (GRASSIC) (1994). Integrated Care for asthma: a clinical, social and economic evaluation. *British Medical Journal* **308**: 559-64

Gregg I and Nunn AJ (1973). Peak expiratory flow in normal subjects. *British Medical Journal* **3**(874): 282-4

Griffiths C, Sturdy P, Naish J et al., (1997). Hospital admissions for asthma in east London: associations with characteristics of local general practices, prescribing, and population. *British Medical Journal* **314**: 482-6

Harding SM (1990) The human pharmacology of fluticasone propionate. *Respiratory Medicine* **84** (suppl A): 25-29

Hargreave F (1988). The drug treatment of asthma: how can it be better applied? *Postgraduate Medical Journal* **64**(suppl 4): 74-81

Hayward SA, Jordan M, Golden G et al., (1996). A randomised controlled evaluation of asthma self management in general practice. *Asthma in General Practice* **4**(2): 11-13

Heeijne den Bak J (1986). Prevalence and management of asthma in children under 16 in one practice. *British Medical Journal* **292**: 175-176

Henry RL, Milner, AD and Davies JG (1983). Simple drug delivery system for use by young asthmatics. *British Medical Journal* **286**: 2021

Hills M and Armitage P (1979). The two period cross over clinical trial. *British Journal of Clinical Pharmacology* **8**: 7-20

Hilton SR (1992). Does patient education work? *British Journal of Hospital Medicine* **47**(6): 438-441

Hilton SR, Sibbald B, Anderson HR et al., (1986). Controlled evaluation of the effects of patient education on asthma morbidity in general practice. *Lancet* **1**: 26-29

Holgate ST (1986). Asthma pathology and the role of inflammatory mediators. *In Childhood Asthma. Update Postgraduate Centre Series.* Sutton, Reed Healthcare Communications, pp 5-12

Holgate ST (1989). The role of inflammatory processes in airway hyper-responsiveness. Report of a meeting at Boca Raton, Florida, USA 3-5 November 1988. *Clinical and experienced Allergy* **19**: 349-65

Holgate ST (1997). The cellular and mediator basis of asthma in relation to natural history. *Lancet* **350**(suppl ii): 5-10

Hoskins G, Neville RG, Smith B et al., (1996). Do self-management plans reduce morbidity in patients with asthma? *British Journal of General Practitioners* **46**(404): 169-171

Hoskins G, Smith B, Neville RG et al., (1998). Tayside Asthma Management Initiative. *Health Bulletin* **56**(2): 586

Hyland ME, Finnis S and Irvine SH (1991). A scale for assessing quality of life in adult asthma sufferers. *Journal of Psychomatic Research* **35**(1): 99-110

Ignacio-Garcia JM and Gonzalez-Santos P (1995). Asthma self-management education program by home monitoring of peak expiratory flow. *American Journal of Respiratory Critical Care Medicine* **151**(2 pt 1): 353-359

International Committee of Medical Journal Editors (1988). Uniform requirements for manuscripts submitted to biomedical journals. *British Medical Journal* **296**: 401-405

Iversen M, Dahl R, Jenson EJ et al., (1989). Lung function and hyperreactivity in farmers. *Thorax* **44**: 645-9

Jenkinson D, Davison J, Jones S et al., (1988). Comparison of effects of a self-management booklet and audio cassette for patients with asthma. *British Medical Journal* **297**: 267-70

Jones A and Sykes AP (1990). The effect of symptom presentation on delay in asthma diagnosis in children in a general practice. *Respiratory Medicine* **84**(2): 139-142

Jones KP, Charlton IH, Middleton M et al., (1993). Targeting asthma care in general practice using a morbidity index. *British Medical Journal* **304**: 1353-6

Jones KP, Mullee MA, Middleton M et al., (1995). Peak flow based asthma self-management: a randomised controlled study in general practice. *Thorax* **50**(8): 851-857

Journal of the Royal College of General Practitioners (1981). Asthma in General Practice. Editorial. **31**: 323-6

Juniper EF, Frith PA and Hargreave FE (1981). Airway responsiveness to histamine and methacholine: relationship to minimum treatment to control symptoms of asthma. *Thorax* **36**: 575-9

Kaur B, Anderson HR, Austin J et al., (1998). Prevalence of asthma symptoms, diagnosis, and treatment in 12-14 year old children across Great Britain (international study of asthma and allergies in childhood, ISAAC UK). *British Medical Journal* **316**: 118 24.

Kelly WJW, Hudson I and Phelan PD (1987). Childhood asthma in adult life: a further study at 28 years of age. *British Medical Journal* **294**: 1059-62

Lahdensuo A, Haahtela T, Herral J et al., (1996). Randomised comparison of guided self management and traditional treatment of asthma over one year *British Medical Journal* **312**: 748-752

Laitinen LA, Naya IP, Binks S et al., (1997). Comparative efficacy of zafirlukast & low dose steroids in asthmatics on prn B2-agonists. *European Respiratory Journal* **10**: (suppl 25) 54(Abstract)

Lancet (1990). Beta-2-agonist in Asthma. Relief, prevention, morbidty. Editorial. **336**: 1411-12

Levy ML (1985). An unusual presentation of childhood asthma [letter]. *Journal of the Royal College of General Practitioners* **35**(281): 590

Levy ML (1986). Delay in diagnosing asthma - is the nature of general practice to blame? (Editorial). *Journal of the Royal College of General Practitioners* **36**(283): 52-53

Levy ML (1988a). Preventable Deaths From Asthma 2: Improving management of severe asthma. *Medical Monitor* **1**(22): 35-36

Levy ML (1988b). Preventable Deaths From Asthma 2: Improving management of severe asthma. *Medical Monitor* **1**(24): 31-32

Levy ML (1994). Royal College of General Practitioners Audit Programme – Asthma Audit: Two recommendations for general practice. *European Respiratory Journal* **7**(suppl 18): 91s

Levy ML (1998). Respiratory diseases: asthma and COPD. In: Garvie DG (Ed) *RCGP Members' Reference Book 1998/9*. pp. 239-243. London, Campden Publishing Ltd

Levy ML and Bell L (1984). General practice audit of asthma in childhood. *British Medical Journal* Clinical Research Ed **289**: 1115-1116

Levy ML, Parmar M, Coetzee D et al., (1985). Respiratory consultations in asthmatic compared with non-asthmatic children in general practice. *British Medical Journal Clinical Research* Ed **291**: 29-30

Levy ML and Hilton SR (1987). *Asthma in Practice*. London, Royal College of General Practitioners

Levy ML, Barnes GR, Howe M et al., (1996). Provision of primary care asthma services in the United Kingdom. *Thorax* **51**: A28 (Abstract)

Levy ML, Barnes GR, Howe M et al., (1998). Asthma Nurse Training Improves Diagnoses in Primary Care. *American Journal of Respiratory and Critical Care Medicine* **157**(3): A633(Abstract)

Levy ML, Robb M, Allen J et al., (1995). Guided self-management reduces morbidity, time off work and consultations for uncontrolled asthma in adults. *European Respiratory Journal* **8**(suppl 19): 318s

Levy ML, Stephenson C and Maslen T (1996). Comparison of short course of oral prednisolone and fluticasone propionate in the treatment of adults with acute exacerbations of asthma in primary care. *Thorax* **51**: 1087-92

Ley P (1976). *In Communications in Medicine.* London, Oxford University Press for the Nuffield Provincial Hospitals Trust

Madge P, McColl J and Paton J (1997). Impact of a nurse led home management training programme in children admitted to hospital with acute asthma: a randomised controlled study *Thorax* **57**(23): 223-228

Maiman LA, Green LW, Gibson G et al., (1979). Education for self treatment by adult asthmatics. *Journal of the American Medical Association* **241**: 1919-22

Majeed A and Moser K (1999). Prescribing for patients with asthma by general practitioners in England and Wales 1994-96. *Health Statistics Quarterly* **1**: 16-20

Majeed A, Evans N and Head P (1997). What can PACT tell us about prescribing in general practice? *British Medical Journal* **315**: 1515-9

Makino S (1966). Clinical severity of bronchial sensitivity to acetyl choline and histamine in bronchial asthma. *Journal of Allergy* **38**: 127-42

Malo J-L, L'Archeveque J, Trudeau C et al., (1996). Should we monitor peak expiratory flow rates or record symptoms with a simple diary in the management of asthma? *Journal of Allergy and Clinical Immunology* **91**(3): 702-9

Malton A, Sumby BS and Dandiker Y (1996). A comparison of in-vitro drug delivery from salbutamol Disks and terbutaline Turbohaler inhalers. *Journal of Pharmaceutical Medicine* **6**(pt 1/3): 35-48

Martin AJ, McLennan LA and Phelan PD (1980). The natural history of childhood asthma to adult life. *British Medical Journal* **280**: 1397-400

Martinez FD (1997). Definition of pediatric asthma and associated risk factors. *Pediatric Pulmonology* **15**(S): 9-12

Martys C (1992). Asthma Care in Darley Dale: general practitioner audit. *British Medical Journal* **304**: 758-60

Mazzuca SA (1982). Does patient education in chronic diseases have therapeutic value? *Journal of Chronic Diseases* **35**(7): 521-29

Melillo G, Cocco G, Balzano et al., (1986) Evaluation of non-specific bronchial hyper reactivity in different respiratory diseases. *European Journal of Respiratory Diseases* **69**(suppl 147): 282-5

McCowan C, Neville RG, Cairns AY et al., (1997). Computer assisted assessment and management of patients with asthma: a preliminary report. pp117-121. BJHC

McFadden ER Jr and Warren EL (1997). Observations on asthma mortality [Review] [93 refs]. *Annals of Internal Medicine* **127**(2): 142-147

McKinley RK, Steele WK (1995). Asthma care in general practice. Letter: comment in *British Medical Journal* **310**: 940-941

Miller M and Levy ML (1997). The role of peak flow meters in asthma care. *Respiratory Disease in Practice* **14**: 16-18

MIMS (1998). London, Haymarket Medical Ltd

Miser WF (1987). Variant forms of asthma. *American Family Physician* **35**(6): 89-96

Mullen PD (1997). Compliance becomes concordance. *British Medical Journal* **314**: 691-692

Naish J, Sturdy P and Toon P (1995). Appropriate prescribing in asthma and its related cost in east London. *British Medical Journal* **310**: 97-100

Neville RG, Hoskins GR, Smith B et al., (1996). Observations on the structure, process and clinical outcomes of asthma care in general practice. *British Journal of General Practice* **46**(411): 583-587

Neville RG (1995). Two Approaches to Effective Asthma Audit. *The Practitioner* **239**: 203-205

Neville RG, Clark RC, Hoskins G et al., (1993). National asthma attack audit 1991-2. *British Medical Journal* **306**: 559-62

Neville RG, Hoskins G, Smith B et al., (1996) Observations on the structure, process and clinical outcomes of asthma care in general practice. *British Journal of General Practice* **46**: 583-7

Neville RG, Hoskins G, Smith B et al., (1997). How general practitioners manage acute asthma attacks. *Thorax* **52**(2): 153-156

Nielsen KG, Auk IL, Bojsen Key et al., (1998). Clinical effect of Disks dry-powder inhaler at low and high inspiratory flow-rates in asthmatic children. *European Respiratory Journal* **11** (2): 350-354

O'Callaghan C and Barry P (1997). Spacer devices in the treatment of asthma. *British Medical Journal* **314**: 1061-1062

Omran M and Russell G (1996). Continuing increase in respiratory symptoms and atopy in Aberdeen school children. *British Medical Journal* **312**: 34

Orr AW (1979). Prodromal itching in asthma. *Journal of the Royal College of General Practice* **29**(202): 287-288

Osman LM, Abdalla MI, Beattie JA et al., (1994). Reducing hospital admission through computer supported education for asthma patients. London, *British Medical Journal*

Osundwa VM and Dawod ST (1989). Vomiting as the main presenting symptom of acute asthma. *Acta Paed Scand* **78**(6): 968-970

Partridge M (1986). Sudden severe asthma. *Respiratory Disease in Practice* **5**: 5-7

Partridge MR (1995). Delivering optimal care to the person with asthma: what are the key components and what do we mean by patient education? *European Respiratory Journal* **8**(2): 298-305

Pearson R (1988). The case for asthma clinics in general practice. *Modern Medicine* **33**: 125-238

Pearson R and Barnes G (1987). Asthma Clinics in general practice: a practice approach. In: Levy M, Ellis and Waine (Ed). Ch 3 pp 15 20. London, RCGP

Pedersen S (1996). Inhalers and nebulisers: which to choose and why. *Respiratory Medicine* **90**: 69-77

Phillips GH (1990) structure-activity relationships of topically active steriods: the selection of fluticasone propionate. *Respiratory Medicine* **84**(suppl A): 19-23

Pinnock H (1996). PACT data analysis – asthma prescribing. *Asthma in General Practice* **4**(1): 5-8

Price DB (1995). Inhaled steroid prescribing over seven years in a general practice and its implications. *European Respiratory Journal* **19**: 463s

Price J (1997). The transition of management from childhood to adolescence. *European Respiratory Review* **7**(40): 19-23

Priel IE (1993). Fatal asthma: where did we go wrong? *Medicine & Law* **12**(3-5): 351-361.

Pringle M and Churchill R (1995). Randomised controlled trials in general practice. *BMJ* **311**: 1382-83

Proceedings of the Asthma mortality task force November 13-16 (1986) (1987). American Academy of Allergy and Immunology and the American Thoracic Society. *Journal of Allergy and Clinical Immunology* **80**(3 pt 2): 361-514

Rafferty P and Holgate ST (1987). Bronchial hyperresponsiveness. In *A New Undertanding in Asthma*. London, Medicom

Rea HH, Scragg R, Jackson R et al., (1986). A case-control study of deaths from asthma. *Thorax* **41**(ii): 833-839

Reiss TF et al., (1998). Montelukast, a once daily leukotriene receptor antagonist in the treatment of chronic asthma: a multi-center, randomised, double-blind trial. *Archives of Intern Medicine* **158**: 1213-1220

Reiss TF, Sorkness CA, Stricker W et al., (1997). Effects of montelukast (MK-0476); a potent cysteinyl leukotriene receptor antagonist, on bronchodilation in asthmatic subjects treated with and without inhaled corticosteroids. *Thorax* **52**(1): 45-48

Rona RJ, Chinn S and Burney PG (1995). Trends in the prevalence of asthma in Scottish and English primary school children 1982-1992. *Thorax* **50**(9): 992-3

Scadding JG (1983). Definition and clinial categories of asthma. In *Asthma*. Ed. Clark TJH and Godfrey S. 2nd ed. London, Chapman and Hall

Scheffer A (1995). Global strategy for asthma management and prevention NHLBI/WHO workshop report. 95-3659, pp.1-176. Bethesda, USA. National Institutes of Health. National Heart, Lung and Blood Institute

Schreier L, Cutler RM and Saigal V (1984). The vomiting asthmatic. *Annals of Allergy* **53**(1): 42-44

Schreier L, Cutler RM and Saigal V (1987). Vomiting as a dominant symptom of asthma *Annals of Allergy* **58**(2): 118-120

Sears MR (1995). Changing patterns in asthma morbidity and mortality. *Journal of Investigational Allergology & Clinical Immunology* **5**(2): 66-72

Seaton A, Godden DJ and Brown K (1994). Increase in asthma: a more toxic environment or a more susceptible environment? *Thorax* **49**(2): 171-4

Sheffer AL and Taggart VS (1993). The national asthma education program. Expert Panel report guidelines for the diagnosis and management of asthma. National Heart, Lung, and Blood Institute. *Medical Care* **31**(3 suppl): MS20-8

Shelley M, Croft P, Chapman S et al., (1996). Is the ratio of corticosteroid to bronchodilator a good indicator of the quality of asthma prescribing? Cross-sectional study linking prescribing data to data on admissions. *British Medical Journal* **313**: 1124 6

Shneerson J (1986). Non-respiratory symptoms of acute asthma. *Thorax* **41**: 701-702

Sibbald B (1992) Genetics. In Asthma: basic Mechanisms and Clinical Management. Ed. Barnes PJ and Thompson NC. 2nd ed. London, Academic press. Pages 21-32

Silverman M (1985). *Asthma in childhood*. London, Current Medical Literature

Silverman MS and Wilson NM (1995). Wheezing disorders in infancy. In: Silverman M (Ed) *Childhood asthma and other wheezing disorders*, pp375-400. London, Chapman Hall

Smith T, Moore EJH and Tunstall Pedoe H (1997). Review by a local medical research ethics committee of the conduct of approved research projects, by examination of patients case notes, consent forms, and research records and by interview. *British Medical Journal* **314**: 1588-90

Speight ANP (1978). Is childhood asthma being under diagnosed and under treated? *British Medical Journal* **2**: 331-2

Speight ANP, Lee DA and Hey EN (1983). Under diagnosis and under treatment of asthma in childhood. *British Medical Journal* **286**: 1253-7

Spelman R (1984). Chronic or recurrent cough in children - a presentation of asthma? *Journal of the Royal College of General Practitoners* **34**(261): 221-2

Spelman R (1991). Two-year follow up of the management of chronic or recurrent cough in children according to an asthma protocol. *British Journal of General Practice* **41**: 406-409

Spelman R (1996). *Guidelines for the diagnosis and management of asthma in general practice*. The Irish College of General Practitioners.

Stableforth DE (1993). Asthma deaths in the United Kingdom. *New Eng & Reg All Proc* **7**(5): 435-438

Staples EB (1991). *British Journal of General Practice*. **41**(347): 232-6

Storr J, Barrell E and Lenney W (1987). Asthma in primary schools. *British Medical Journal* **295**: 251-2

Strachan DP (1995a). Epidemiology. In: Silverman A (Ed) *Childhood asthma and other wheezing disorders*, pp7-31. Chapman and Hall, London.

Strachan DP (1995b). Epidemiology of hay fever: towards a community diagnosis. *Clinical and Experimental Allergy* **25**(4): 296-303

Strachan DP, Anderson HR, Bland JM et al., (1988). Asthma as a link between chest illness in childhood and chronic cough and phlegm in adults. *British Medical Journal* **296**: 890-3

Strachan DP, Golding D and Brown K (1990). Regional variations in wheezing illness in British children: effect of migration during early childhood. *Journal of Epidemiology and Community Health* **44**(3): 231-6

Strachan DP, Anderson HR, Limb ES et al., (1994). A national survey of asthma prevalence, severity, and treatment in Great Britain. *Archives of Diseases in Childhood* **70**(3): 174-8

Suissa S, Dennis R, Ernst P et al., (1997). Effectiveness of the leukotriene receptor antagonist zafirlukast for mild-to-moderate asthma. A randomized, double-blind, placebo-controlled trial. *Annals of Internal Medicine* **126**(3): 177-183

Swinscow T (1983). *Statistics at Square One*. London, BMA

The British Thoracic Society Nebuliser Project Group Standards of Care Committee (1997). Current Best Practice for nebuliser treatment. *Thorax* **52**(suppl 2): S1-3

The British Thoracic Society, The National Asthma Campaign, The Royal College of Physicians of London, The General Practitioner's in Asthma Group, The British Association of Accident and Emergency Medicine, The British Paediatric Respiratory Society and The British Paediatric Association (1997). The British Guidelines on Asthma Management: 1995 Review and Position Statement. *Thorax* **52**(suppl 1): S1-S21.

The COPD Guidelines Group of the Standards of Care Committee of the BTS (1997). BTS Guidelines for the management of chronic obstructive pulmonary disease. *Thorax* **52**(5): S1-S28

The International Study of Asthma and Allergies in Childhood (ISAAC) Steering Committee (1998). Worldwide variation in prevalence of symptoms of asthma, allergic rhinoconjuctivitis, and atopic eczema: ISAAC. *Lancet* **351**: 1225-32

Toop LJ (1985) Active approach to recognising asthma in general practice. *British Medical Journal* **290**: 1629-1631

Townsend J, Wilkes H, Haines A et al., (1991). Adolescent smokers seen in general practice: Health, lifestyle, physical measurements and response to anti-smoking advice. *British Medical Journal* **303**: 947-950

Tsanakas JN, Bannister OM, Boon AW et al., (1986). The peak flow whistle: a simple device for monitoring peak flow in children. *British Medical Journal* **293**: 1410

Tudor Hart J (1970). Semicontinuous screening of a whole community for hypertension. *Lancet* **2**: 223-226

Tudor Hart J (1986). Wheezing in young children: problems of measurement and management. *Journal of the Royal College of General Practice* **36**(283): 78-81

Usherwood TP and Barber JH (1988). Audit of process and outcome in a mini-clinic for children with asthma. *Family Practice* **5**(4): 289-93

Van der Palen J, Klein JJ, Zielhuis GA et al., (1998). The role of self-treatment in self-management education for adult asthmatics. *Respiratory Medicine* **92**: 668-675

Von Mutius E, Fritzch C, Weiland SW et al., (1992). Prevalence of asthma and allergic disorders among children in united Germany: a descriptive comparison. *British Medical Journal* **305**: 1395-9

Wardman AG, Binns V, Clayden AD et al., (1986). The diagnosis and treatment of adults with obstructive airways disease in general practice. *British Journal of Diseases of the Chest* **80**(1): 19-26

Ware JH, Ferris BG, Dockery DW et al., (1986). Effects of ambient sulfur oxides and suspended particles on respiratory health of pre-adolescent children. *American Review of Respiratory Diseases* **133**(5) 834-42

Whincup PH, Cook DG, Strachan DP et al., (1993). Time trends in respiratory symptoms in childhood over a 24 year period. *Archives of Diseases in Childhood* **68**(6): 729-34

White PT, Pharoah CA, Anderson HR et al., (1989). Randomised controlled trial of small group education on the outcome of chronic asthma in general practice. *Journal of the Royal College of General Practitioners* **39** :182-6

Williams H and McNicol KN (1969). Prevalence, natural history and relationship of wheezy bronchitis and asthma in children. An epidemiological study. *British Medical Journal* **iv**(679): 321-5

Wilson SR, Scamagas P, German DF et al., (1993). A controlled trial of two forms of self management education for adults with asthma. *American Journal of Medicine* **94**(6): 564-576

Woolcock AJ, Peat JK, Salome CM et al., (1987). Prevalence of bronchial hyperresponsiveness and asthma in rural adult population. *Thorax* **42**: 361-8

Yen K, Salome C and Woolcock AJ (1983). Rapid method for measurement of bronchial responsiveness. *Thorax* **38**: 760-5

Yoon R, McKenzie DK, Bauman A et al., (1993). Controlled trial evaluation of an asthma education programme for adults. *Thorax* **48**(ii): 1110-1116

INDEX